THE SHAPE OF SPACE

FOOD PREPARATION SPACES

THE SHAPE OF SPACE

FOOD PREPARATION SPACES

CRANE · DIXON

VNR VAN NOSTRAND REINHOLD
_____ New York

Acknowledgements

The authors wish to extend their thanks to the following individuals, companies and institutions who kindly assisted with the preparation of this book.

Graham Barrie and Christopher Nutt of Berkeley Food Equipment for providing a considerable amount of technical data, which was particularly relevant for the chapter on commercial kitchens.
Disabled Foundation, Royal National Institute for the Blind and the Institute for the Partially Sighted for their assistance.
Chris King for his neat and eloquent drawings.
Last, but by no means least, we must thank our colleague Nenad Lorencin who has undertaken the bulk of the detailed research and compilation of this book.

Published in the United States of America by
Van Nostrand Reinhold
115 Fifth Avenue
New York, New York 1003

Distributed in Canada by
Nelson Canada
1120 Birchmont Road
Scarborough, Ontario M1K 5G4, Canada

16 15 14 13 12 11 10 9 8 7 6 5 4 3 2 1

FOREWORD

This book is intended as a tool for architects, interior designers and other professionals to identify the space requirements for domestic or commercial kitchens and food preparation areas. The size and shape of kitchens are often determined by external factors rather than the internal operating requirements.

The various factors of access, servicing and function, combined with the often predetermined size and shape make many food preparation areas unique. The purpose of this book is to identify the principles applying in various situations and to show by example how the same basic functional criteria can be satisfied within a variety of spatial contexts.

The book is divided into five chapters dealing with domestic and commercial kitchens, food serveries and foods courts and retail catering. Each chapter identifies the various criteria to be borne in mind when preparing layouts, and provides specimen plans and information that can be applied directly to a wide range of food preparation facilities.

In preparing this book we have consciously intended the information to be plagiarized or copied directly, either by photocopying, cutting and pasting, tracing or computer scanning. All the images are drawn to scale and can be used same size or resized as required. Our aim has been to provide information that will enable the designer to identify design parameters and our examples provide possible schematic solutions.

In conclusion it should be noted that catering design is an extensive and highly specialized subject. This book concentrates on dimensional criteria and internal function relationships and is intended to generate ideas more than solving all problems.

Detailed technical and statutory requirements such as public health regulations and servicing have not been covered in this book.

The book has been prepared by architects in designing and implementing catering facilities and whilst every endeavor has been taken to ensure the information is correct, the book is not intended to supplant or replace the experienced catering consultant or design company.

CONTENTS

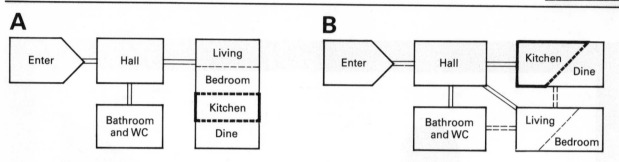

A

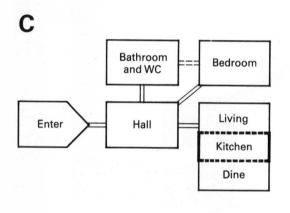

B

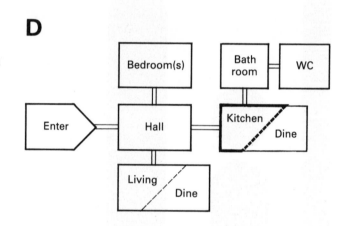

C

D

E

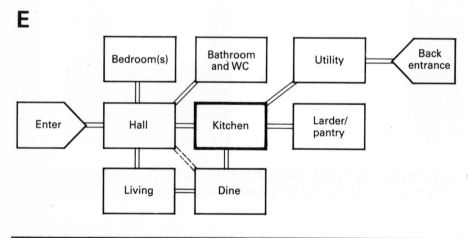

NTS

A   Example of a studio: kitchen is part of living
    accommodation; lobby to WC required.
B   Example of a studio/1 bedroom apartment: kitchen
    and dining areas combined.
C   Example of a 1 bedroom apartment: kitchen
    combined with living and dining areas.
D   Example of a 1/2 bedroom apartment: bathroom
    off kitchen/dining areas, acting as a lobby to WC.
E   Example of a 2+ bedroom house: centralized
    kitchen with access to front and back entrances.

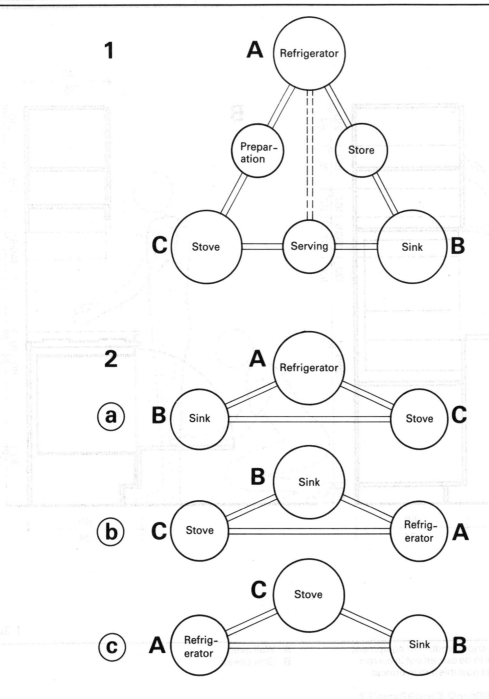

NTS

- The total length of the work triangle should average between 6.5m/*21'8"* and 7.0m/*23'4"*.
- Through circulation is to be kept away from the work triangle and should not cross the sink (B) to stove (C) route.
- The sink to stove is the most used route. It should be between 1.2m/*4'* and 1.8m/*6'*.

1	Work flows.
1A	Refrigerator/larder: electricity supply required.
1B	Sink and drain: window above sink advisable; water supply and drain required.
1C	Stove: extract exhaust above cooker; electricity and gas required.
2	Work centers.
2A	Refrigerator.
2B	Sink.
2C	Stove.

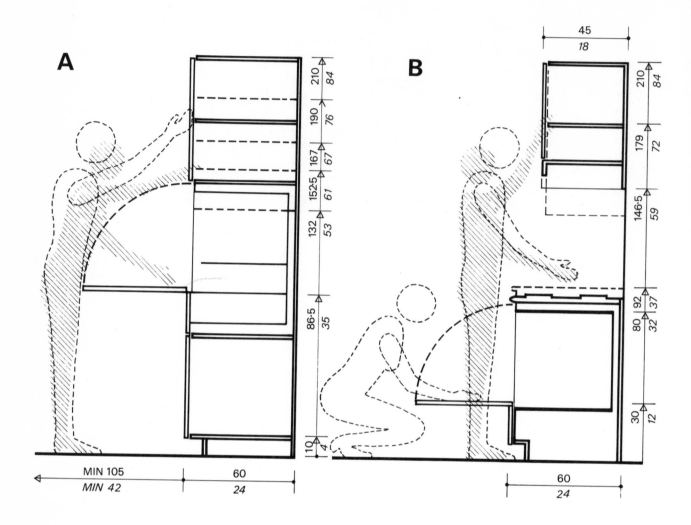

A

210	84
190	76
167	67
152·5	61
132	53
86·5	35

MIN 105
MIN 42

60
24

B

45
18

210	84
179	72
146·5	59
92	37
80	32
30	12

10 | 4

60
24

1:20

- Dimensioning – height, depth, width – of equipment for operations and work to be carried out in correct ways, with minimum toil possible and in utmost safety.
- Stove height between 800mm/*2′8″* and 920mm/*3′1″* (people taller than 1.8m/*6′* require top of equipment to be higher than 920mm/*3′ 1″*.

- Heavy goods should be stored at a low level or waist height.
- Light goods/equipment should be stored above shoulder height.
- Minimum 1.8m²/*9ft.²* of space is required for basic storage with an additional 0.5m²/*5ft.²* per person served.
- High level units with a narrower depth for easier access to the back of units are used in preparation.
- For washing-up, if possible, the sink should be situated by a window for natural light, thus avoiding units over. Alternatively, artificial light below a high level unit is required (body creating own shadow). 2m/*6′8″* and 1.8m/*6′″*.

A Wall oven.
B Stove/oven.

C Storage.
D Preparation.
E Washing up.

(Illustrations are shown on **1.04**)

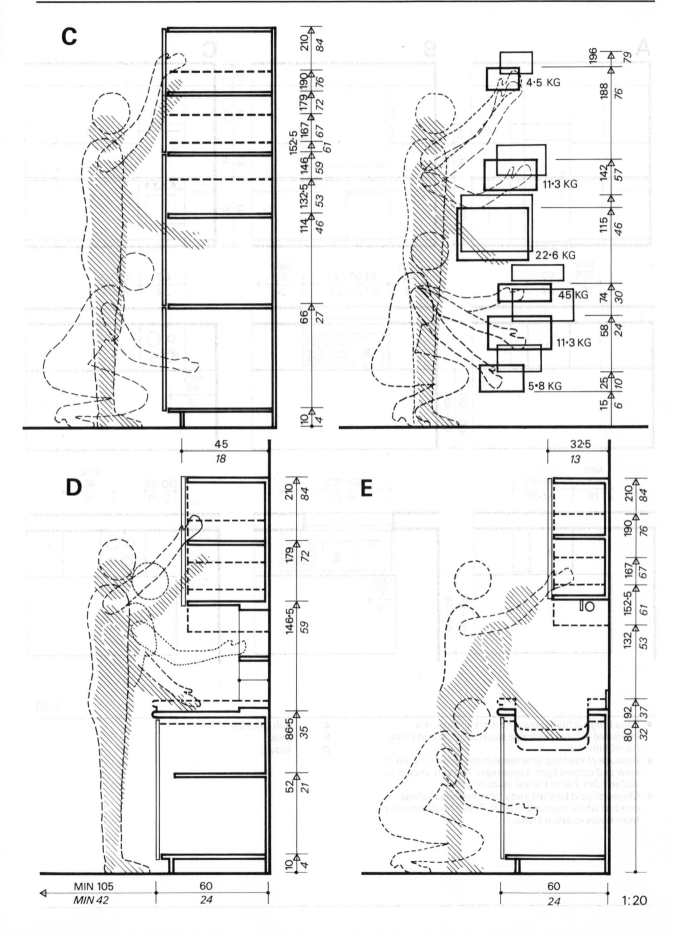

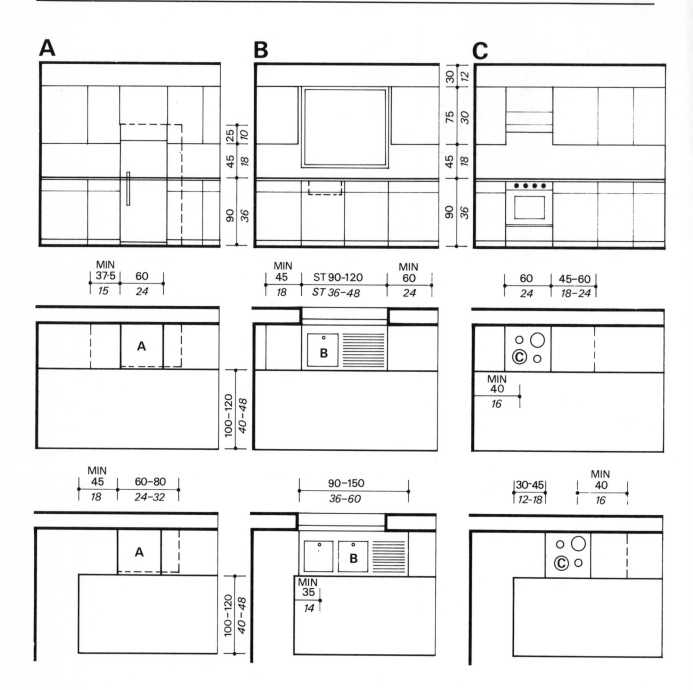

1:50

- If the fridge is higher than the work surface, it is advisable to have the fridge situated at the end of the run of fitments.
- Because of the long time spent in the wash-up zone, a view and natural light is necessary. The sink should be within 2.3m/7'0" of the soil stack or gulley.
- Stoves should be sited away from corners to allow comfort whilst standing in front. They should be away from doors to avoid drafts.

A   Refrigerator.
B   Sink.
C   Stove.

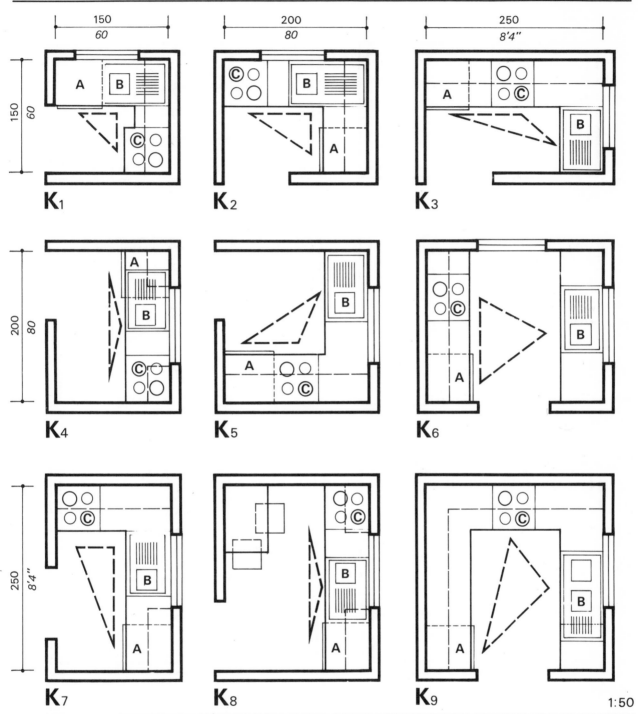

K_1 K_2 K_3

K_4 K_5 K_6

K_7 K_8 K_9

1:50

- The layouts shown are samples based on studies of furniture, appliances, storage and clearances for average residential kitchens.
- Sizes vary from 2.25m²/21ft.² (e.g. studio, 1 person) to 12.25m²/122ft.² (4 bedroom house, 6–8 persons).

Note: Long light dashes indicate high-level units over. Heavy long dashes indicate work flow.

A	Refrigerator.
B	Sink.
C	Stove.
K1, K2	"L" shaped for 1–2 persons (minimum dimensions).
K3	"L"-shaped for 1–2 persons.
K4	Single wall for 1–2 persons (minimum dimensions).
K5	"L"-shaped for 1–2 persons.
K6	Parallel wall for 2–3 persons.
K7	"L"-shaped for 1–2 persons.
K8	Single wall for 1–2 persons.
K9	"U"-shaped for 2–3 persons.

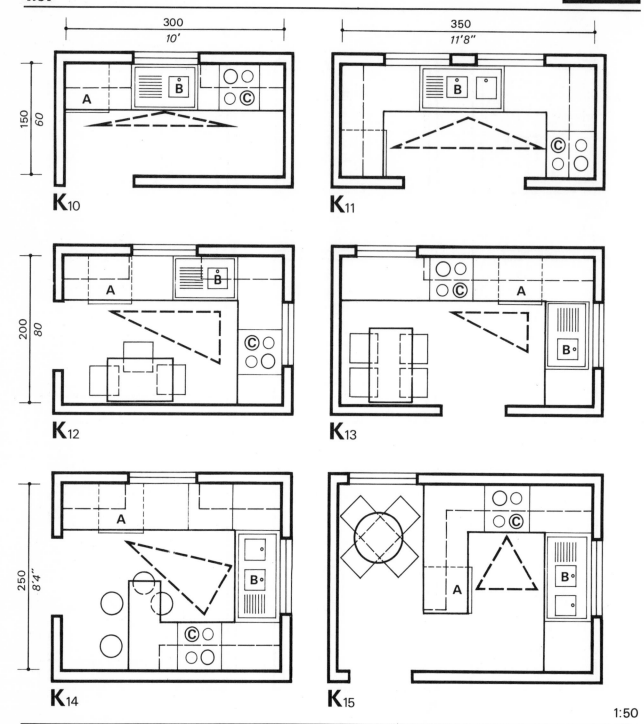

1:50

- Further examples of single wall, "U"-shaped and "L"-shaped kitchens.

A	Refrigerator.
B	Sink.
C	Stove.
K10	Single wall for 1–2 people.
K11	"U"-shaped, pantry type for 1–2 people.
K12, K13	"L"-shaped for 3–4 people.
K14	"U"-shaped with breakfast bar for 3–4 people.
K15	"U"-shaped with dining area for 3–4 people.

1.08

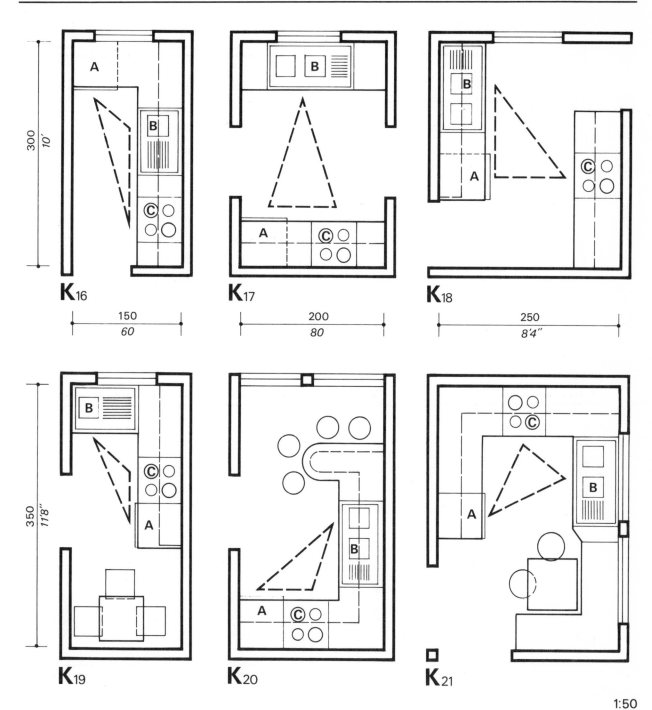

1:50

- Further example of "L"-shaped, parallel wall and "U"-shaped kitchens.

A	Refrigerator.
B	Sink.
C	Stove.
K16	"L"-shaped for 2–3 people (fridge a long way from entrance).
K17, K18	Parallel wall for 2–4 people (through circulation is a disadvantage).
K19	"L"-shaped for 2–3 people (small eating area).
K20	"L"-shaped for 3–4 people (breakfast bar).
K21	"U"-shaped for 4–5 people (built-in breakfast/dining area).

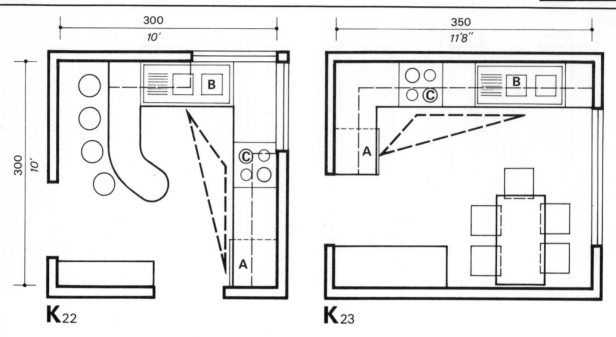

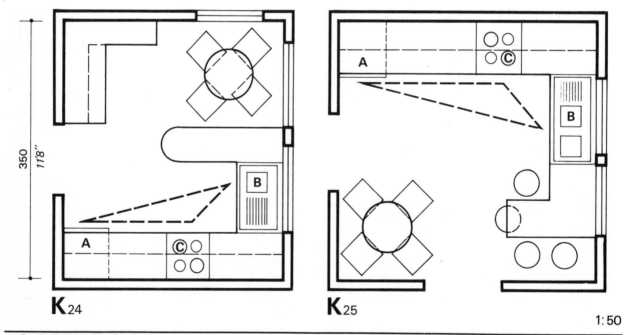

1:50

- Further examples of "L"-shaped and broken "U"-shaped kitchens.

A   Refrigerator.
B   Sink.
C   Stove.
K22   "L"-shaped for 4–6 people (through circulation avoids work circulation area and breakfast bar).
K23   "L"-shaped for 4–6 people (large dining area, therefore separate dining room could be omitted).
K24   Broken "U"-shape for 4–6 people (dining area).
K25   "L"-shaped for 6–8 people (breakfast bar and dining area).

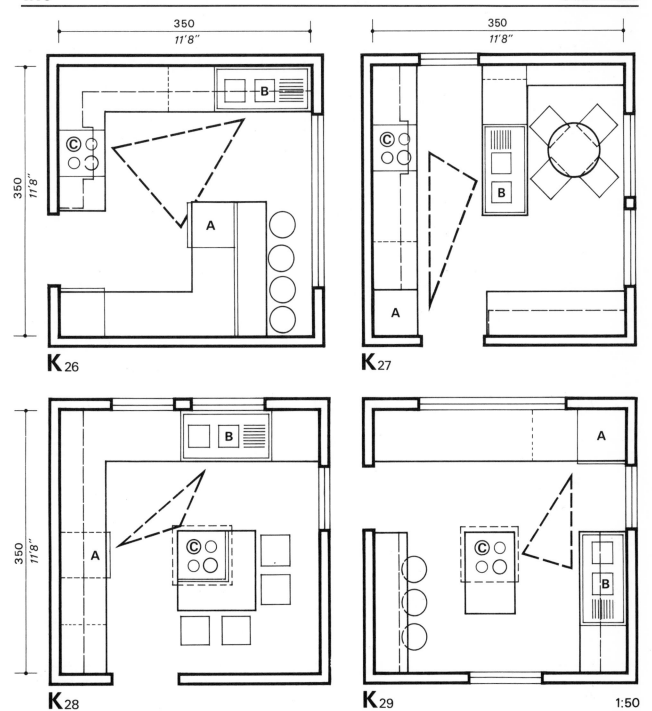

K26

K27

K28

K29

1:50

● Examples of kitchens in which one of the work stations (refrigerator, stove or sink) is located in the center of the kitchen.

A Refrigerator.
B Sink.
C Stove.
K26 Broken "U" for 6–8 people (centralized refrigerator, with adjacent breakfast bar).
K27 Parallel wall for 6–8 people (centralized sink with dining area).
K28 "L"-shaped for 6–8 people (centralized stove and breakfast bar).
K29 Broken "L" for 6–8 people (centralized stove).

1.11

A

B

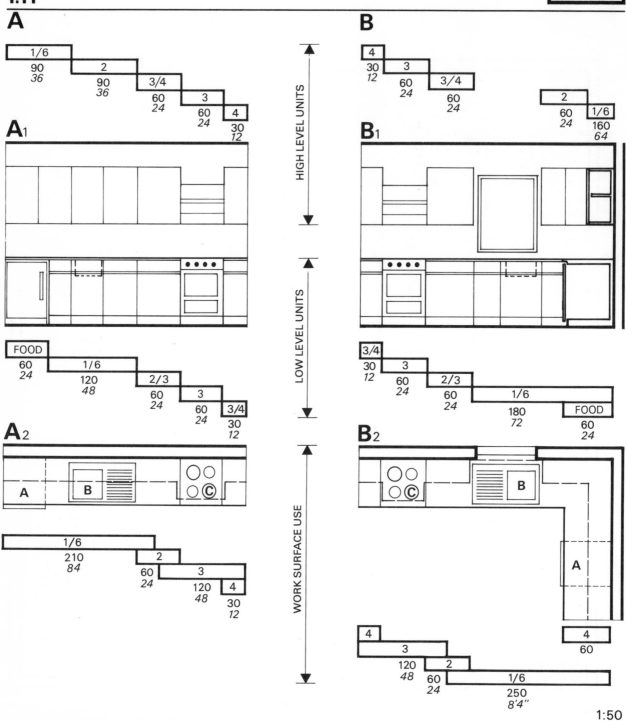

A₁

B₁

HIGH LEVEL UNITS

LOW LEVEL UNITS

WORK SURFACE USE

A₂

B₂

1:50

(For details of activity sequence see 1.12.)

- Working assembly is made up of basic meal preparation zones, sometimes incorporating eating space. Zones may be arranged in a straight line, but walking distances can be reduced and space better used forming "L" or "U" shapes.
- Direction of workflow is a matter of choice, but may depend on the position of exterior plumbing stacks, doors, windows, etc.
- USA practice: right to left sequence.
  European practice: left to right sequence.
- Worktops should not be less than 300mm/12" wide.

A Straight line working zone.
A1 Elevational view of straight line working zone.
A2 Plan view of straight line working zone.
B "L"-shaped working zone.
B1 Elevational view of "L"-shaped working zone.
B2 Plan view of "L"-shaped working zone.

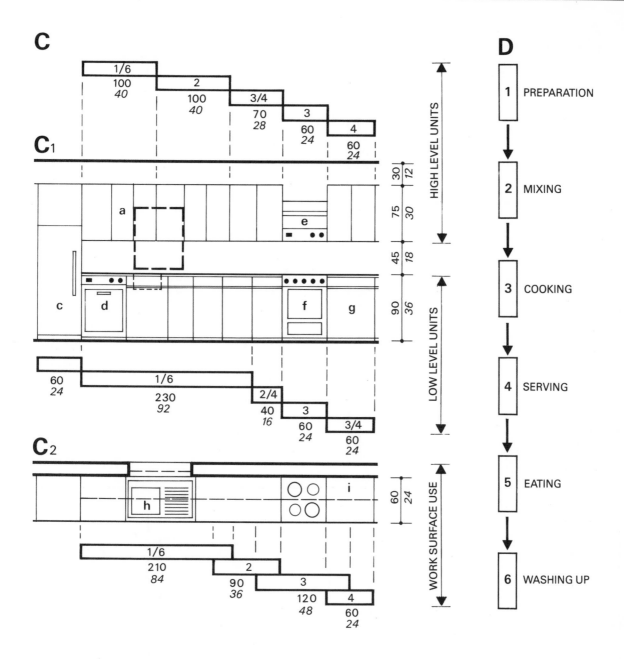

1:50

- Simplest example of single-line, 4-person assembly with possible variations. (Window over sink would displace some wall storage in preparation/wash-up zone.) Total storage shown in this example is the minimum recommended for households of 3 or more people in local authority housing.
- Adjacent activity zones may share a common length of worktop. Additional 300mm/12" to shared counter would cover both counters.
- **a** High level storage.
- **b** Suggested window position.
- **c** Fridge.
- **d** Dishwash machine.
- **e** Cooker head.
- **f** Cooker.
- **g** Low level storage units.
- **h** Sink and drain.
- **i** Worksurface.

C Straight line working zone.
C1 Elevational view of straight line working zone.
C2 Plan view of straight line working zone.
D Activity sequence.
D1 Preparation: Includes unwrapping, washing, peeling, chopping and mincing.
D2 Mixing: Includes weighing, measuring and mixing.
D3 Cooking: Includes baking, boiling, frying and grilling.
D4 Serving: Includes keeping food hot and putting food into dishes.
D5 Eating: Includes table laying, eating and clearing.
D6 Washing-up: Includes disposing of waste, stacking, washing/drying and putting away.
Note: Heavy dashes indicate window instead of high-level cupboards.

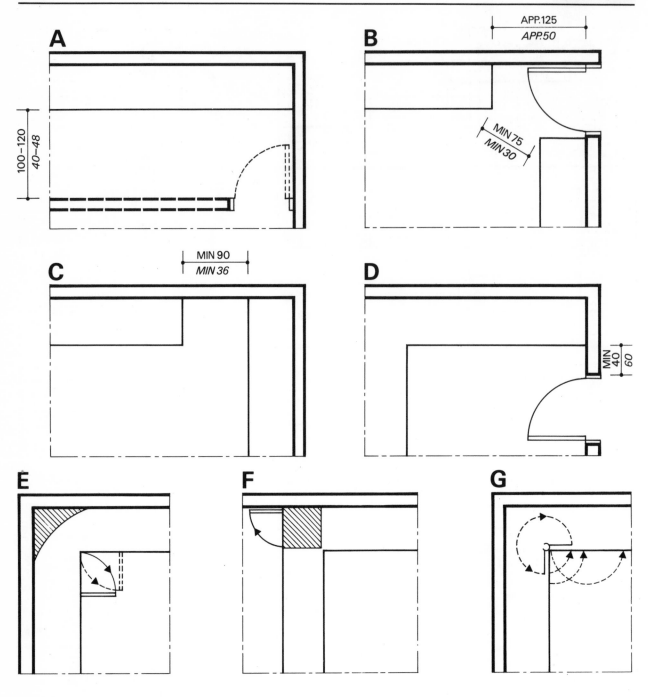

1:50

A–D Minimum clearances between fittings, walls and work surfaces, and doors and work surfaces. If door is nearer to work surface than 400mm/*1'6"* (diagram D), outward opening door should be used. Diagram B arrangement is not recommended but may be unavoidable.

E Shows zone below counter difficult to reach.

F, G Give two options for optimum use of space. Care is needed to prevent clashing doors at corners.

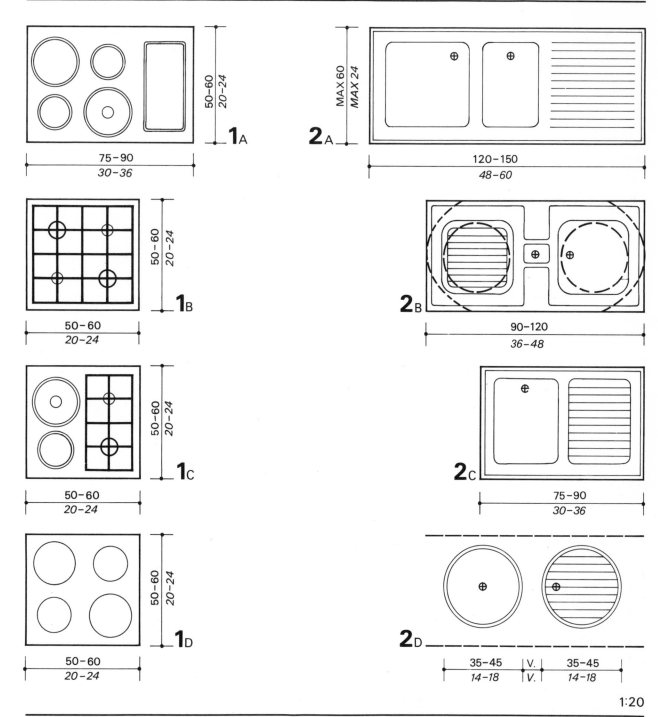

1:20

1	STOVES	**2**	SINKS
1A	Electric automatic plates with large hot plates.	**2A**	Double sink with drainer.
1B	Gas elements with varying heat intensity.	**2B**	Recessed sink and drain with central waste
1C	Combination gas and electric stove.		disposal (enamel, earthenware or stainless steel).
1D	Glass ceramic top with temperature zones marked	**2C**	Compact sink with drain or double sink – recessed
	(easy maintenance).		or full worktop width.
		2D	Individual recessed sinks.

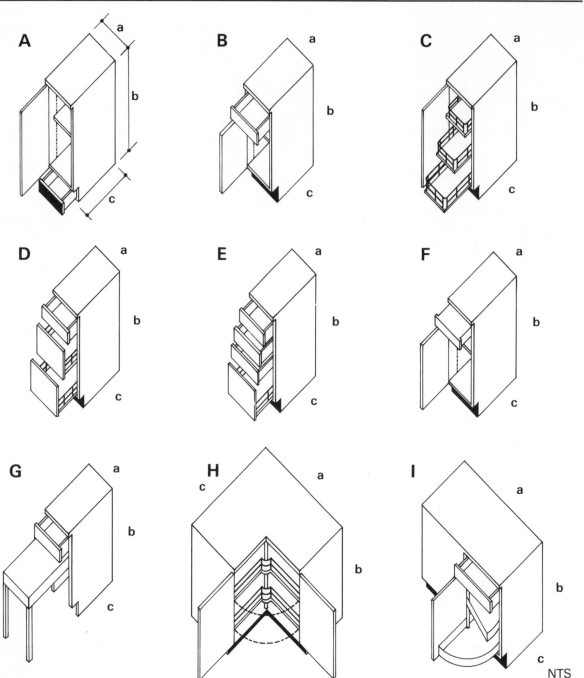

- Permanent fittings vary in size and comprise worktop storage shelves and kick plate base, constructed from plywood or similar. Finish should be hard wearing (e.g. plastic veneer).
- Internal shelves to be covered in linoleum, plastic or metal. Low units are used for heavier goods such as equipment.

A Standard 600×600mm/*24"×24"* low level unit with pull out plinth shelf.

B Top drawer on ball bearings and height adjustable shelf.

C Three height adjustable wire basket pull-outs on rails with ball bearings.

D Top drawer and 2 individual pull-outs with wire baskets.

E Three drawers and pull-out wire basket.

F Pull-out table 300mm/*12"* as extended work surface 800mm/*32"* high.

G Pull-out table on legs, 600mm/*24"* extension, 700mm/*28"* high.

H Corner unit with three-quarter circle carousel, two turning levels. Door opens 180°.

I Corner unit with two semi-circular carousels which can be turned individually.

	a (width)	b (height)	c (depth)
A, B, C, D, E	30–60cm/ *12"–24"*	80–90cm/ *32"–36"*	50–60cm/ *20"–24"*
F, G	30–60cm/ *12"–24"*	80–90cm/ *32"–36"*	60cm/*24"*
H	100cm/*40"*	80–90cm/ *32"–36"*	50–60cm/ *20"–24"*

A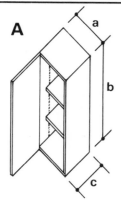

B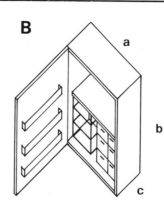

C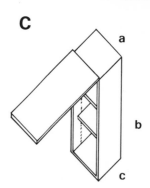

D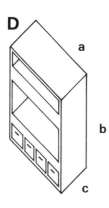

E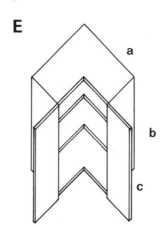

F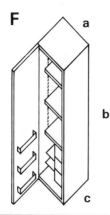

G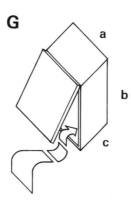

NTS

• High level storage units (wall mounted) are usually shallow to allow use of work top below and to allow access to top shelves.

A Standard unit with shelves.
B Unit with 6 containers and spice racks.
C Unit with lifting door.
D Open unit with shelves and drawers.
E Corner wall unit with 180° doors.
F Higher unit/extra storage.
G Self operating extractor when the flap door is opened.

	a (width)	b (height)	c (depth)
A, B, C, D	30–60cm/12″–24″	75cm/30″	30–60cm/12″–24″
E	60cm/24″	75–105cm/30″–42″	60cm/24″
F	30–60cm/12″–24″	105cm/42″	30cm/12″

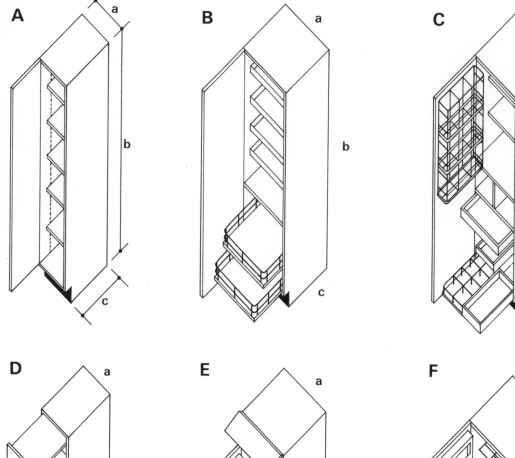

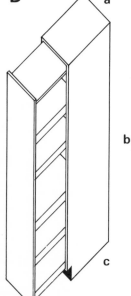

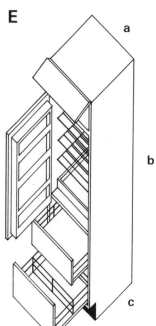

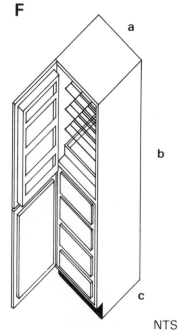

NTS

- Tall storage units could serve as broom cupboards or pantries/larders or may contain an eye level fridge.
- Refrigerators/freezers are sometimes encased to match remaining units.

A Standard tall unit with inlay shelves.
B Storage unit with drawers, wire basket pull-outs and inlay shelves.
C Storage unit with pull-out drawers and wire frame bottle rack.
D Pull-out storage unit with full length front door.
E Tall unit for fridge with top box and pull-out drawers.

	a (width)	b (height)	c (depth)
A, B, C,	30–60cm/ *12"–24"*	200cm/*80"* max	50–60cm/ *20"–24"*
D	30–45cm/ *12"–18"*	200cm/*80"* max	50–60cm/ *20"–24"*
E, F	50–60cm/ *20"–24"*	200cm/*80"* max	50–60cm/ *20"–24"*

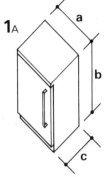

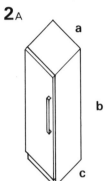

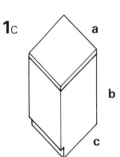

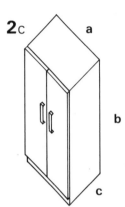

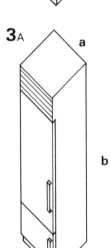

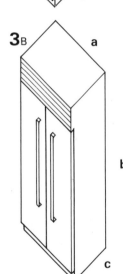

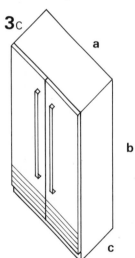

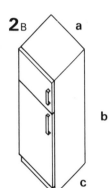

- The user has to bend to have full access to standard (under-counter refrigerators/freezers.
- Door opening swing clearances should be considered when laying out a kitchen (door as wide as refrigerator).

1	Standard (under-counter) refrigerators/freezers to fit below work surface.
1A	Single door (interior freezer).
1B	Side by side.
1C	Top loading (freezer only).
2	Standard (high).
2A	Single door (interior freezer).
2B	Top freezer (separate freezer).
2C	Side by side (separate freezer).
3	Built-in high.
3A	Bottom freezer (separate freezer).
3B	Side by side (separate freezer).
3C	Combination (separate freezer).

	a (width)	b (height)	c (depth)
1A	60cm/*24"*	88cm/*36"*	50–60cm/ *20"–24"*
1B	60–90cm/ *24"–36"*	88cm/*36"*	50–60cm/ *20"–24"*
1C	60–150cm/ *24"–60"*	88cm/*36"*	60–80cm/ *24"–32"*
2A	50–60cm/ *20"–24"*	140–160cm/ *56"–64"*	50–60cm/ *20"–24"*
2B	60–84cm/ *24"–34"*	140–170cm/ *56"–68"*	60–80cm/ *24"–32"*
2C	78–90cm/ *32"–36"*	140–175cm/ *56"–70"*	60–80cm/ *24"–32"*
3A	60–90cm/ *24"–36"*	180+30cm/ *72"+12"*	60–90cm/ *24"–36"*
3B	90–120cm/ *36"–48"*	180+30cm/ *72"+12"*	60–90cm/ *24"–36"*
3C	120–180cm/ *48"–72"*	180–210cm/ *72"–84"*	60–90cm/ *24"–36"*

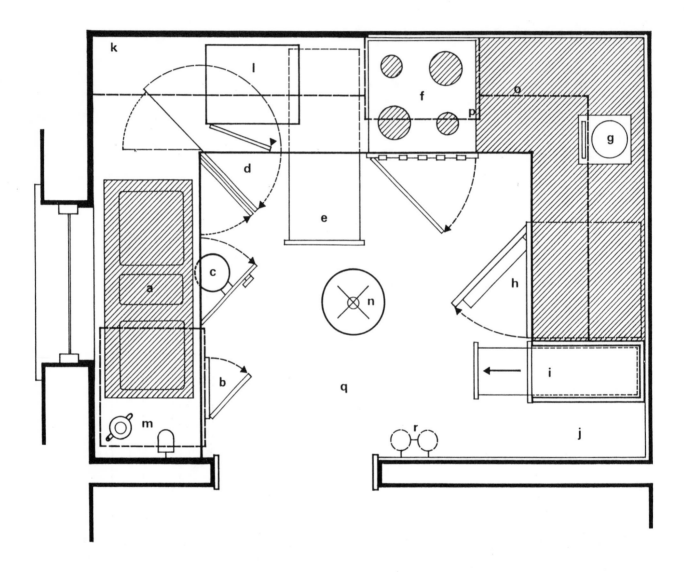

1:20

- Lighting should be bright with spotlights over the stoves, sink and worktops. Dimmer switches are required. Fluorescent strip lighting should be used as the general lighting.
- Controls to the stove, microwave and washing machine should have dimpled/profiled markings.
- Storage jars and handles should be in bright colors.

a Sink and drain in dark enamel (contrasting to cooker).
b Washing machine below sink.
c Refuse bin on back of door, opened by a peddle.
d Corner unit with semi-circular carousel, maximising storage.
e Pull-out table/work top.
f Corner and convector oven (electric).
g Talking scales
h Refrigerator below dark worktop.
i High pull-out storage unit.
j Ironing board, brooms storage.

k White worktop with contrasting dark tiles on walls.
l Microwave.
m Tea making area with high level tea dispenser.
n Adjustable height stool.
o Shelves over, preferably without doors (sliding if necessary). Storage jars should be in different colors and sizes.
p Cooker hood over cooker.
q Non-slip floor.
r H/L fire extinguisher and blanket.

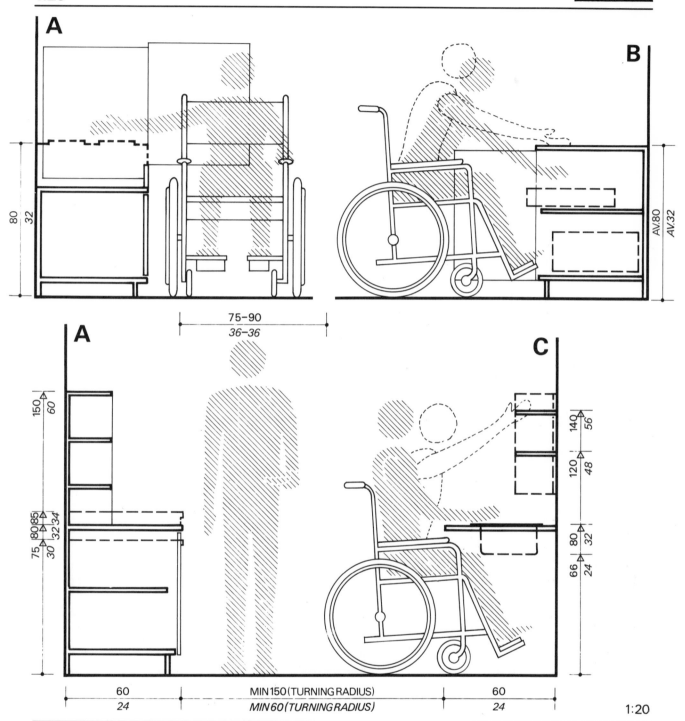

75–90
36–36

60 / *24*   MIN 150 (TURNING RADIUS) / *MIN 60 (TURNING RADIUS)*   60 / *24*

1:20

- Smooth non-skid floor surface is required (linoleum or vinyl).
- Stove top controls are at the front of the appliance to avoid reaching across hot surfaces.
- Side by side refrigerator/freezer is preferred.
- Dishwashers should be front loading.
- Vertical drawers in base cabinets/or sliding pull outs on ball bearings allow for access to out of reach areas.

A Stove.
B Storage.
C Wash-up.

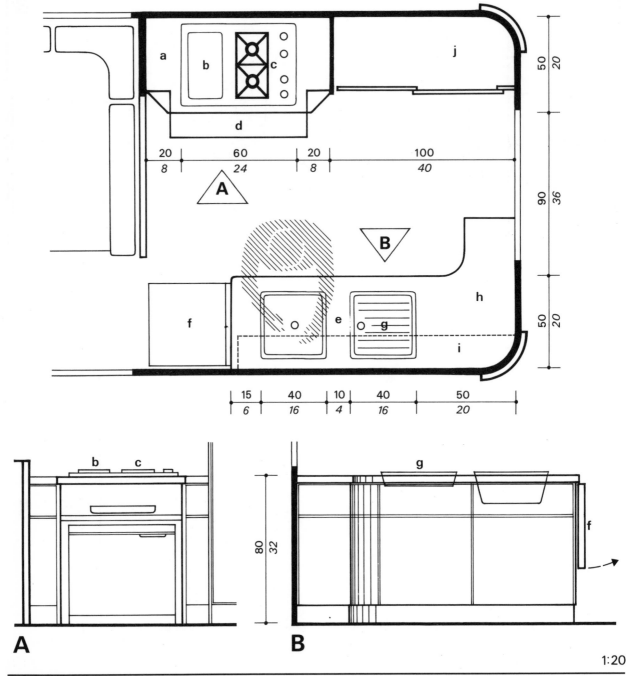

A

B

1:20

- Example of motor home kitchenette (taken from Renault caravan). Minor deviations to widths but length and layout will differ.
- **a** Extract exhaust hood over.
- **b** Electric hotplate.
- **c** Gas rings.
- **d** Fridge and grill under.
- **e** Storage under.
- **f** Hinged worktop.
- **g** Sink drainer.
- **h** Worktop.
- **i** Shelves under.
- **j** Wardrobe.

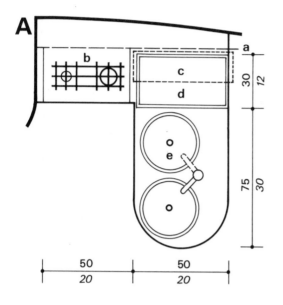

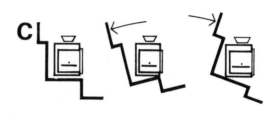

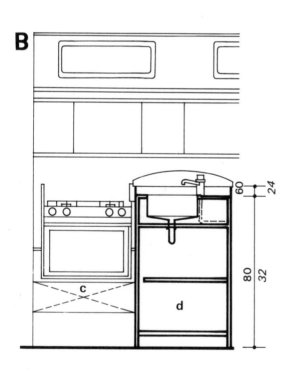

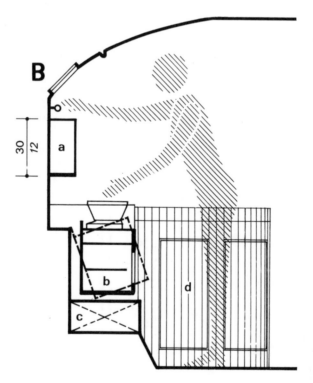

1:20

A Plan view of yacht galley.
B Sectional view of yacht galley.
C Gimballs The stove stays in the vertical position.
Note: This is an example of a galley with minimum sizes to maximise space (30ft sailing boat for 6 persons). Larger boats have galleys similar to domestic kitchens.

a Line of cupboard over.
b Gas stove.
c Sliding tray.
d Inset tray.
e 350° stainless steel sink.
f Cupboard.
g Oven range.
h Gas store.
i Storage.

DOMESTIC FOOD PREPARATION
Circulation of air, heat and fumes

1.23

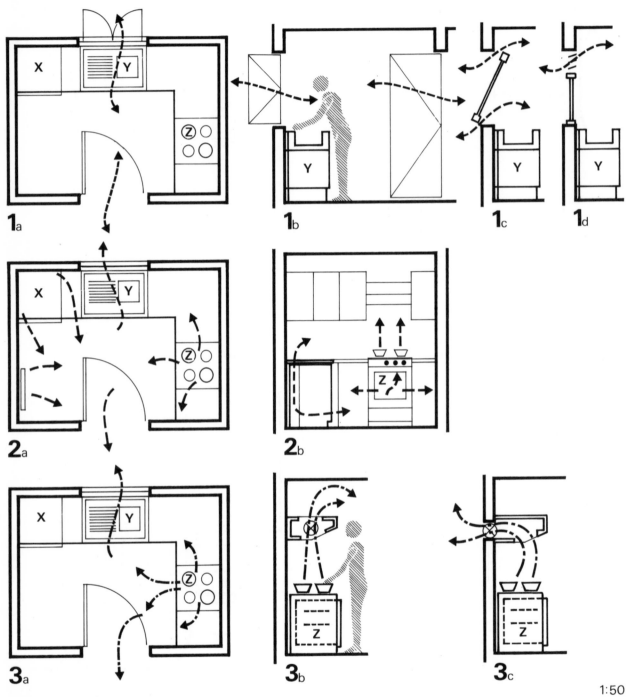

1:50

A	Plan view of circulation of air, heat and fumes through a kitchen.
B	Sectional view of ciculation of air, heat and fumes through a kitchen.
X	Refrigerator.
Y	Wash-up.
Z	Stove.

1	Air
1a, 1b	Air movement through open windows and doors.
1c	Tilting windows allow good circulation.
1d	Louvres allow constant air circulation preventing condensation.
2	Heat
2a, 2b	Heat radiates from sides and top of cooker and over and radiators (if installed). Kitchen radiators are usually not required.
3	Fumes
3a	Flames from cooking ascend.
3b	Mechanical hood cleans air within hood and recirculates it into kitchen.
3c	Air is extracted to outside.

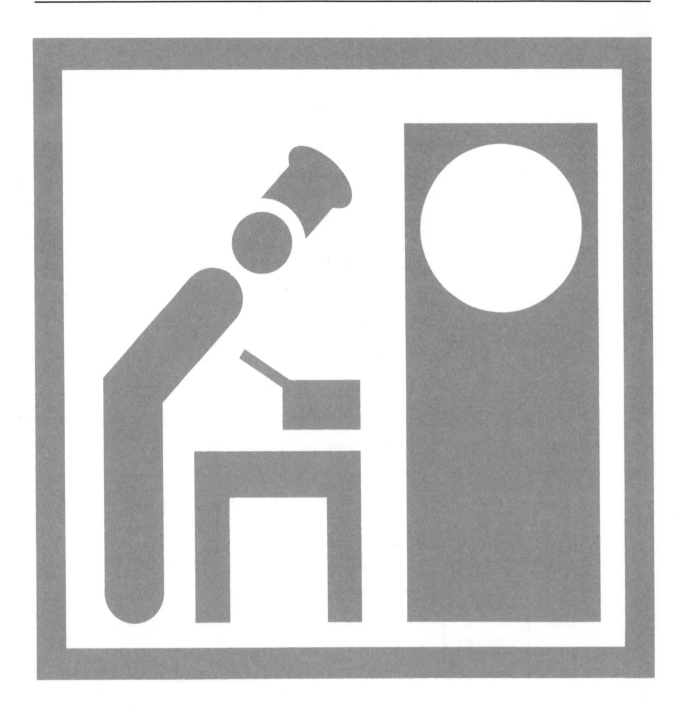

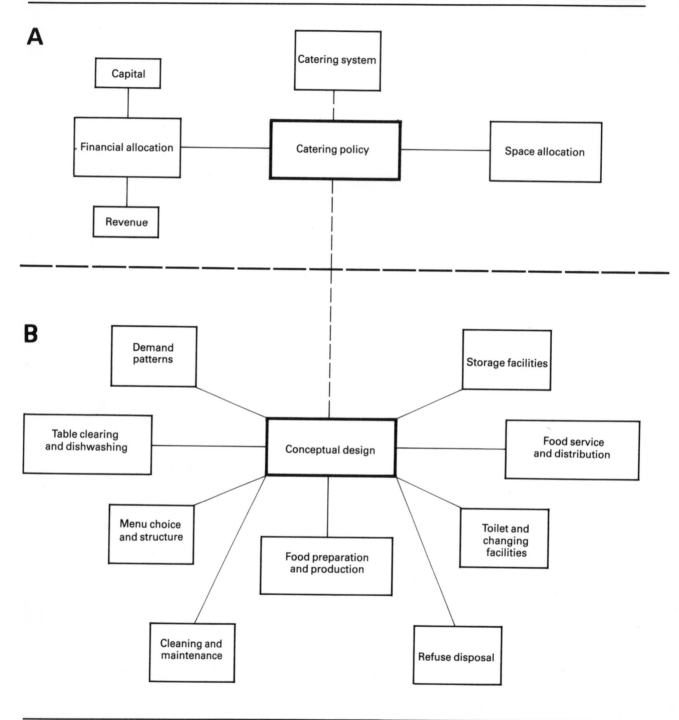

A

Catering system

Capital

Financial allocation

Catering policy

Space allocation

Revenue

B

Demand patterns

Storage facilities

Table clearing and dishwashing

Conceptual design

Food service and distribution

Menu choice and structure

Toilet and changing facilities

Food preparation and production

Cleaning and maintenance

Refuse disposal

A Feasibility of project.
B Design considerations.

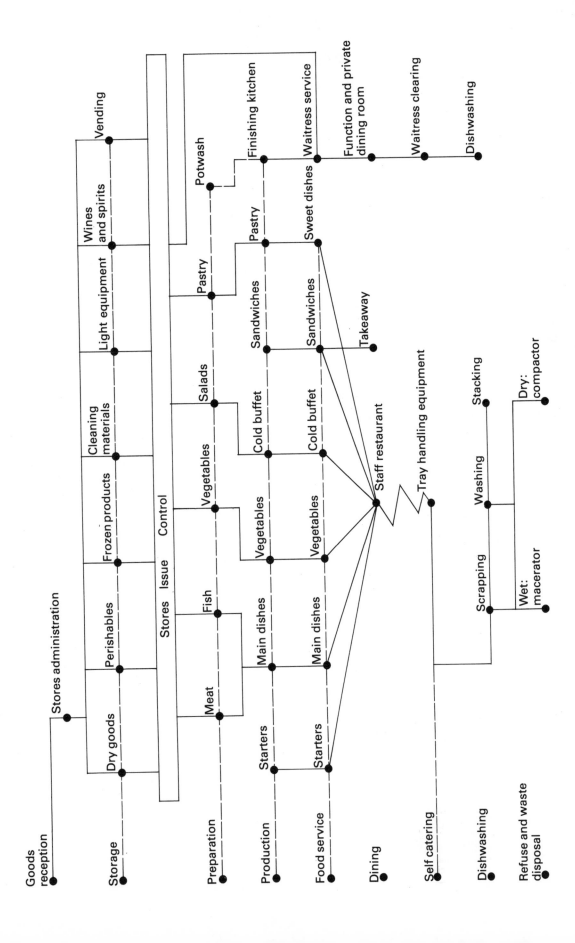

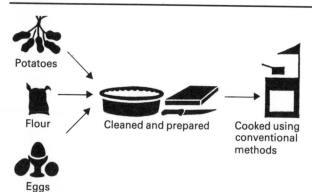

Potatoes

Flour

Cleaned and prepared

Cooked using conventional methods

Eggs

1 Conventional

The production process involves the purchase of raw materials in their natural state. The raw materials are then prepared and cooked using conventional cooking equipment.

The use of pure conventional methods is normally limited to high quality commercial restaurants and directors dining rooms, where budgets and tariffs can support the additional skilled labour and space costs.

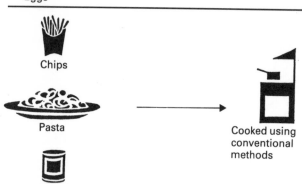

Chips

Pasta

Cooked using conventional methods

Tinned stew

2 Conventional/convenience

This production process is the format currently employed by most staff restaurants and midrange commercial facilities. The process involves the use of preprepared raw materials together with a range of mixes and semi and fully prepared menu items.

The use of this system allows the caterer to maximise output whilst limiting labour, equipment and space costs.

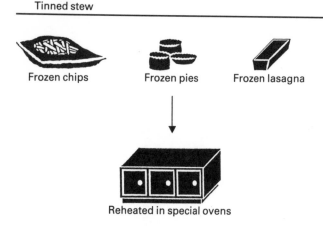

Frozen chips

Frozen pies

Frozen lasagna

Reheated in special ovens

3 Cook/chill

This process is based upon the use of menu items which are pre-prepared and pre-cooked in a central production kitchen. The food is chilled once the cooking and portioning process has been completed and can be held for up to 5 days at 0°C to 3°C, including the day of production and the day of service.

The pre-cooked food in then re-generated (re-heated) in specially designed ovens immediately prior to service.

The system has the effect of reducing the space required in the kitchen area, but the servery, dining and dishwashing areas are unaffected.

Labour costs are also reduced as less staff are required to prepare the food for service.

The greatest benefits of the system are enjoyed where evening and weekend services are required for which premium labour rates are paid or where a number of catering facilities within a limited area can be provided from a production unit. The system has been most cost effective in hospitals and large factory sites.

Careful feasibility studies should be carried out before the system is adopted as initial capital costs can be high and saving low if the basic criteria are not met.

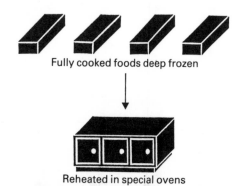

Fully cooked foods deep frozen

Reheated in special ovens

4 Cook freeze

The same basic principles apply with this process as for cook chill. However, the use of cook freeze allows greater flexibility in storage and transport as storage is not limited to 5 days and frozen products are more robust and less liable to damage in transport.

A major problem included in cook freeze is that many products deteriorate dramatically and cannot be refrozen, so that that range and scope of menu items is reduced unless complex preparation and production methods are used.

The system is normally adopted where transport problems occur or in conjunction with cook chill.

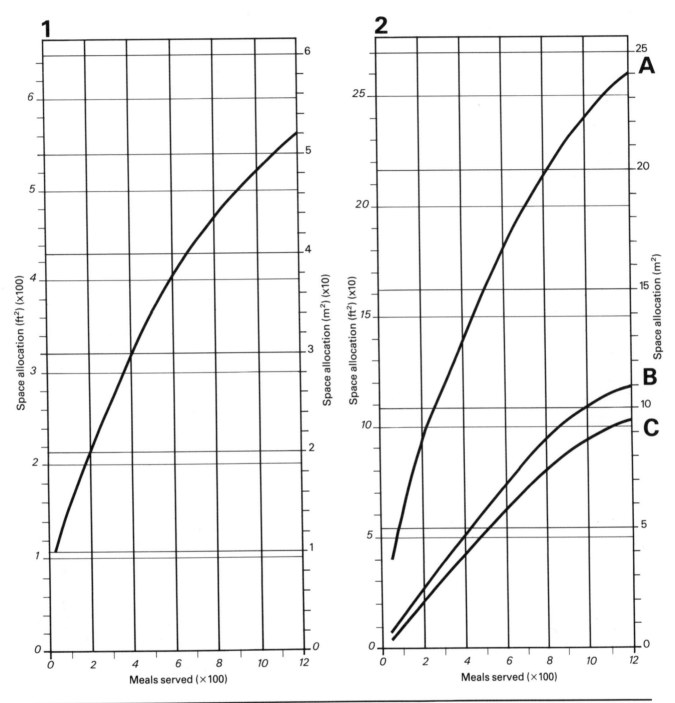

1 The above graph shows total storage areas for dry, refrigerated and cleaning materials only. Other areas such as liquor, linen and light equipment should be considered individually, frozen as necessary, depending upon the type of operation.

2 Graphs to show space allocation for different types of storage.
A Dry storage
B Refrigerated from 0°C to 3°C *(32°F to 36°F)*.
C Frozen from −18°C to −21°C *(−0.4°F to −5.8°F)*.

A

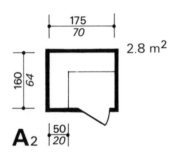

A_1

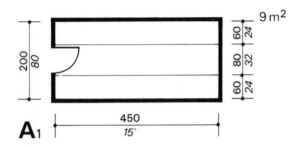

A_2

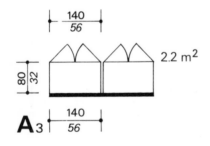

A_3

B

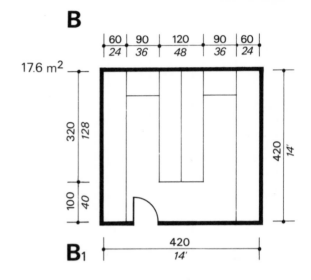

B_1

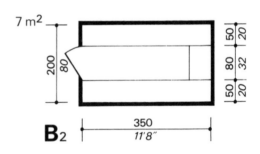

B_2

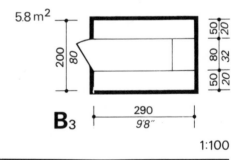

B_3

1:100

A1, B1 Dry stores.
A2, B2 Refrigerated stores from 0°C to 3°C *(32°F to 36°F)*.
A3, B3 Deep freeze stores from −18°C to −21°C *(−0.4°F to −5.8°F)*.
(See 2.06)

A Layout of dry stores, refrigerated stores and deep freeze stores for 200 meals.

B Layout of dry stores, refrigerated stores and deep freeze stores for 600 meals.

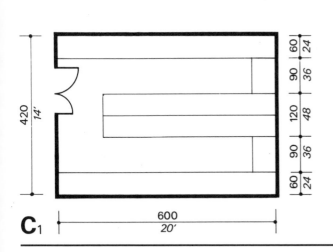

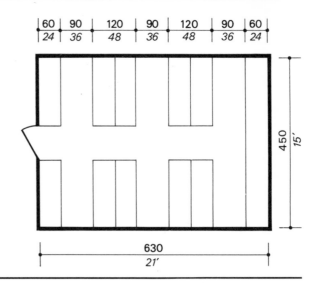

C1

C2

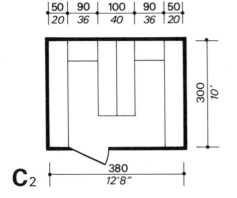

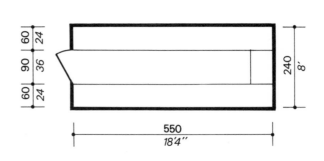

C3

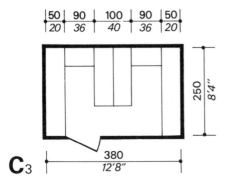

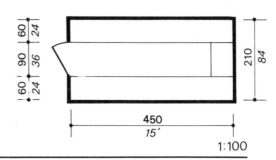

1:100

- Dry stores: The options show optimum widths of rooms to maximize linear storage per square meter.
- Refrigerated stores: Enclosures are normally modular and formed in 75mm/3" thick panels. In smaller kitchens refrigerated cabinets could replace cold room enclosures.
- Deep freeze stores: Enclosures are also formed in 75mm/3" thick panels. An insulated floor is required to avoid damage to the structural floor. In smaller kitchens freezer cabinets can be used.

C1 Layout of dry stores for 1200 meals.
C2 Layout of refrigerated stores for 1200 meals.
C3 Layout of deep freeze stores for 1200 meals.

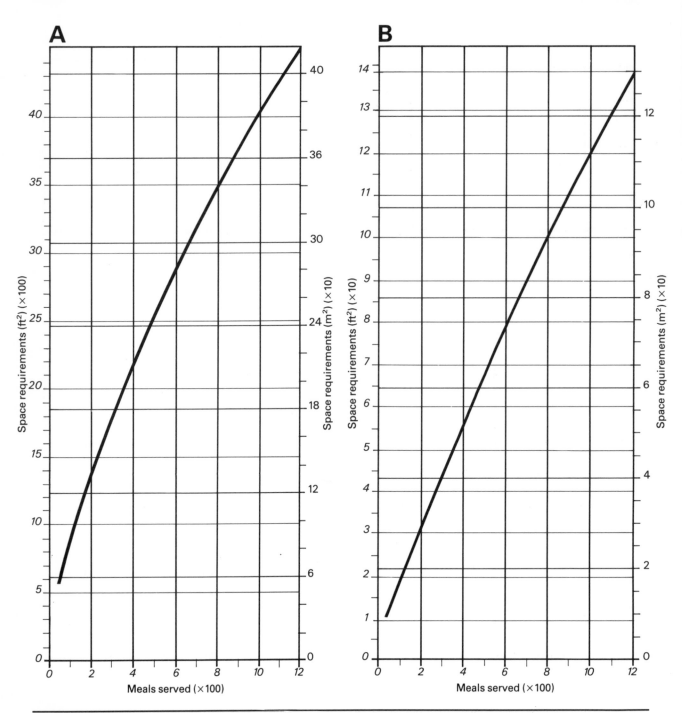

- The space allocations should be regarded as a guide and not definitive as factors such as menu choice and the shape of the space available will affect the overall figures.
- Food service areas are normally based upon the free flow principle where numbers in excess of 200 are served. The system splits the normal straight line counter into a number of separate units, each serving a different dish, to divide demand and minimize potential lines.

A Graph to show overall space requirements.
B Graph to show service space requirements

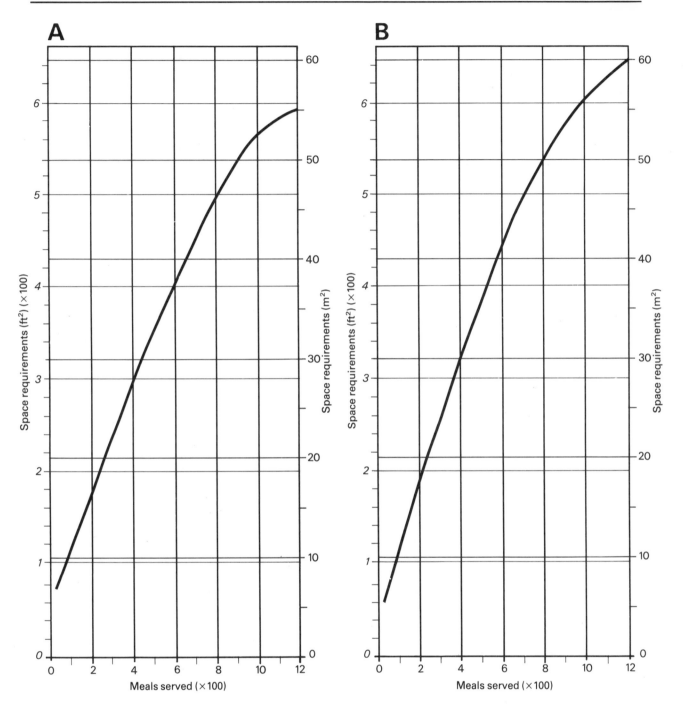

- In smaller kitchens the preparation areas are normally not defined and surround the production area to minimize walking distances. In larger kitchens, areas are designated and normally split into main dish, vegetable/salad and pastry areas.
- In smaller kitchens the production equipment is usually set against a wall rather than island sited. However, this normally occurs in kitchens serving up to 200 meals or where areas dictate.

A Graph to show space requirements for preparation.
B Graph to show space requirements for production.

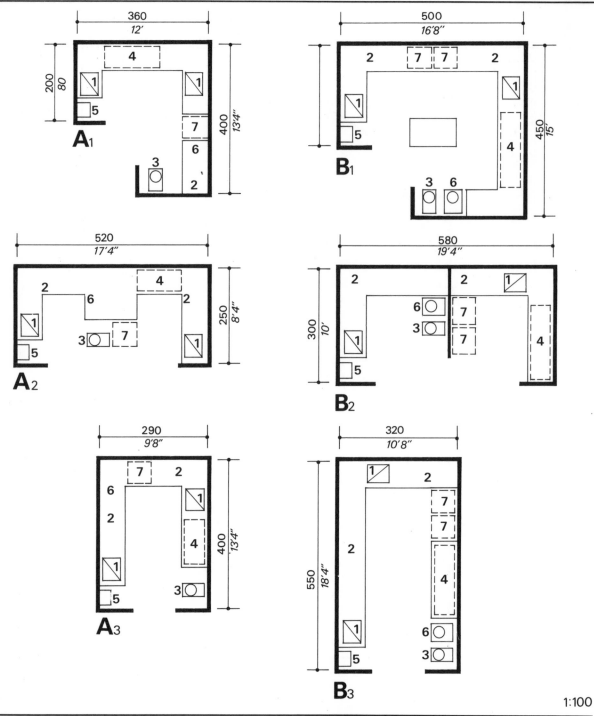

A1, A2, A3 Examples of layouts for 600 meals.
B1, B2, B3 Examples of layouts for 1200 meals.

1 Sink unit.
2 Preparation bench.
3 Mixing machine.
4 Refrigeration.
5 Wash hand basin.
6 Food processor.
7 Multitier rack.

1:100

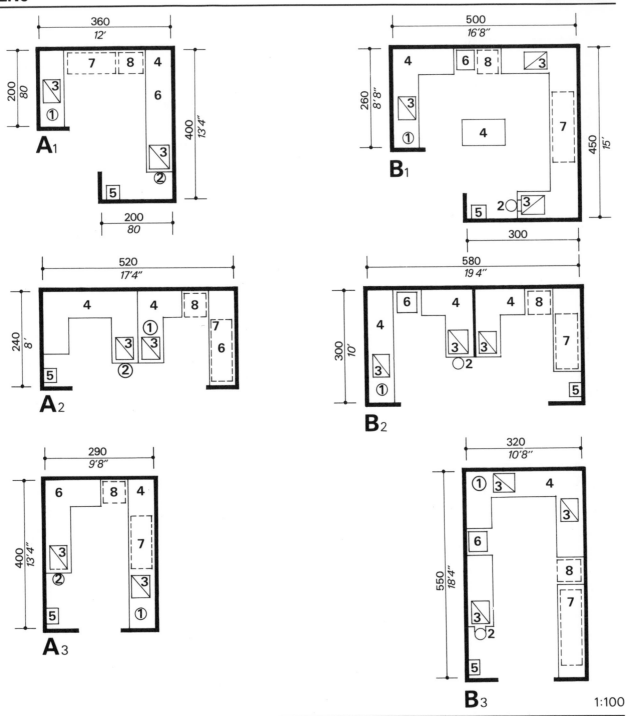

1:100

1 Waste disposal.
2 Potato peeler.
3 Sink unit.
4 Bench unit.
5 Wash hand basin.
6 Vegetable preparation.
7 Refrigeration.
8 Multitier trolley.

A1, A2, A3 Examples of layouts for 600 meals.
B1, B2, B3 Examples of layouts for 1200 meals.

Options
● Wall shelving.
● Wall cupboards.
● Salad washer.

The use of potato peelers and vegetable preparation
machines is dictated by the caterer as all products can be
bought in a preprepared form if required.

COMMERCIAL FOOD PREPARATION
Layouts for pastry preparation and production:
600 and 1200 meals

2.11

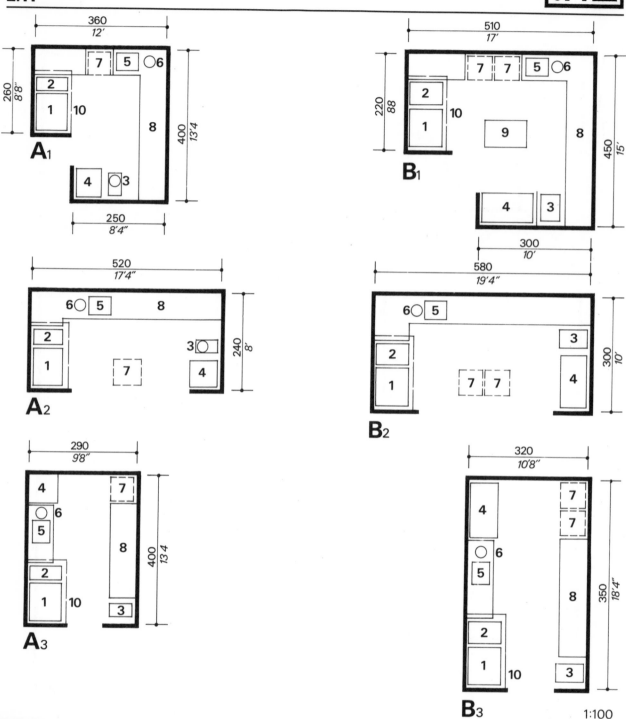

1:100

A1, A2, A3 Examples of layouts for 600 meals.
B1, B2, B3 Examples of layouts for 1200 meals.

1 Two-tier convection oven.
2 Two-ring boiling top.
3 Food mixer.
4 Roll-in refrigerator.
5 Sink unit.
6 Wash hand basin.
7 Multitier racks.
8 Bench unit.
9 Mobile table.
10 Extractor/exhaust canopy.

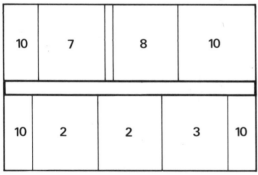

A

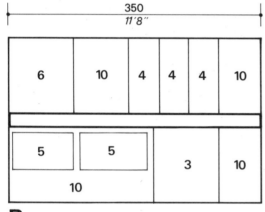

B₁

C₁

B₂

C₂

1:50

A	Example of a layout for 200 meals.
B1, B2	Examples of a layout for 600 meals.
C1, C2	Examples of a layout for 1200 meals.

1 Bratt pan, 600mm/*24"*.
2 Bratt pan, 900mm/*36"*.
3 Oven range.
4 Deep freeze.
5 Salamander.
6 Combination oven.
7 Combination oven.
8 Convection oven, 1 tier.
9 Convection oven, 2 tier.
10 Lay-off bench.

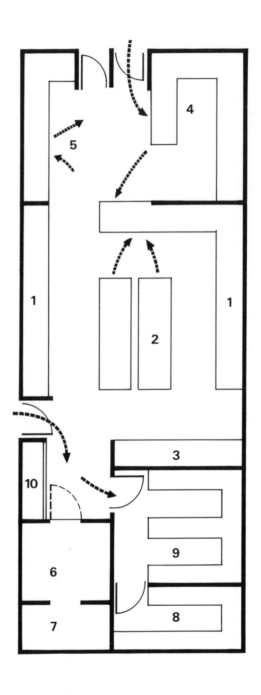

1:100

Note. Administration offices and staff wash and changing rooms are not shown.
Total area is 96m².

1 Preparation.
2 Production.
3 Potwash.
4 Dishwash.
5 Waiting pantry.
6 Cold room.
7 Deep freeze.
8 Dry store.
9 Liquor store.
10 Cleaning materials.

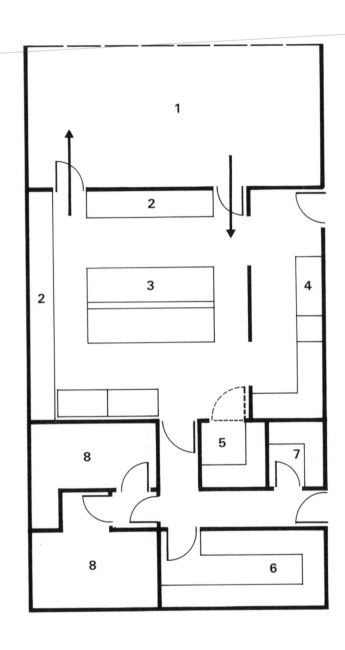

1:100

Note 1. For serving area information, see Section 3.
Note 2. For typical room layouts, see analysis sheets.
Note 3. Administration office has not been included in
the space allocation or layout.
Total area is 120m².

1 Serving area.
2 Preparation.
3 Production.
4 Dishwash/Potwash.
5 Cold room.
6 Dry stores.
7 Cleaning materials.
8 Washroom and changing.

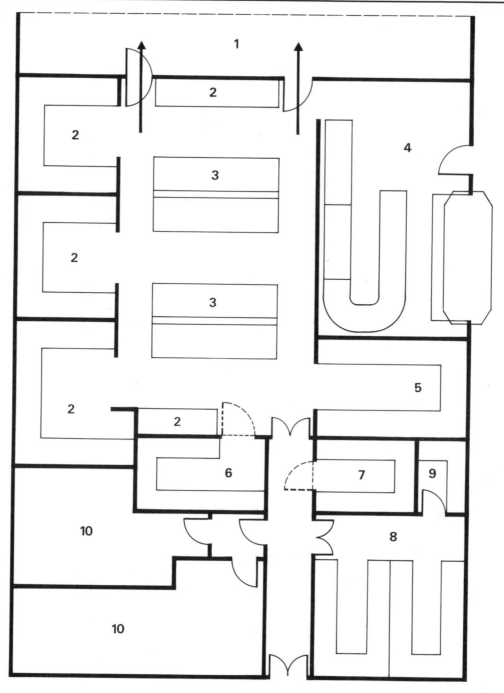

1:100

Note 1. For serving area information see Section 3.
Note 2. Administration and chef's office (if required) have
not been included in the space allocation or layout.

1 Serving area.
2 Preparation.
3 Production.
4 Dishwash.
5 Potwash.
6 Cold room.
7 Deep freeze.
8 Dry stores.
9 Cleaning materials.
10 Washroom and
changing.

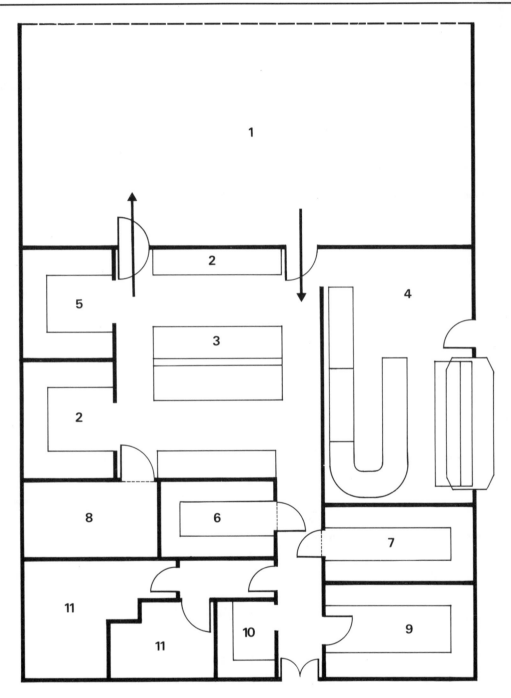

1:100

Note 1. For serving area information see Section 3.
Note 2. Administration offices have not been included in the layout.

1 Serving area.
2 Preparation.
3 Production/regeneration.
4 Dishwash.
5 Potwash.
6 Cold room.
7 Deep freeze.
8 Holding cold room – delivered finished product.
9 Dry stores.
10 Cleaning materials.
11 Washroom and changing.

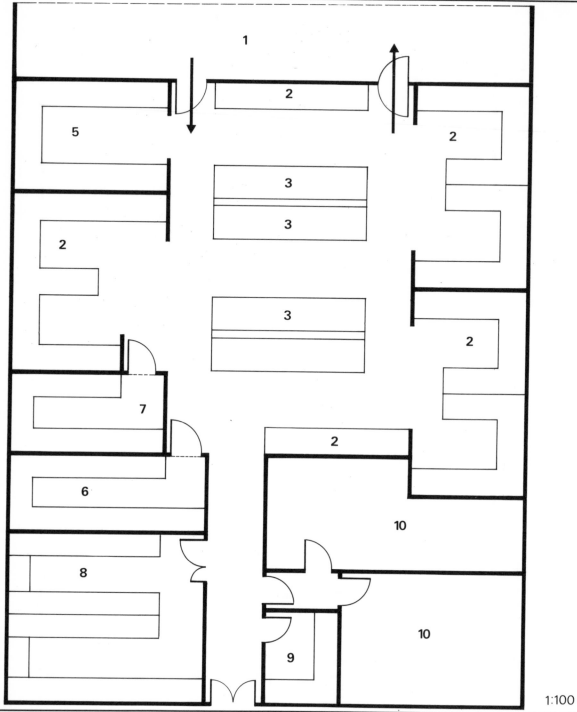

1:100

Note 1. For serving area information, see Section 3.
Note 2. Administration and chef's offices have not been
included in the layout.

1 Serving area.
2 Preparation.
3 Production.
4 Dishwash – remote
   location.
5 Potwash.
6 Cold room.
7 Deep freeze.
8 Dry store.
9 Cleaning materials.
10 Washroom and
    changing.

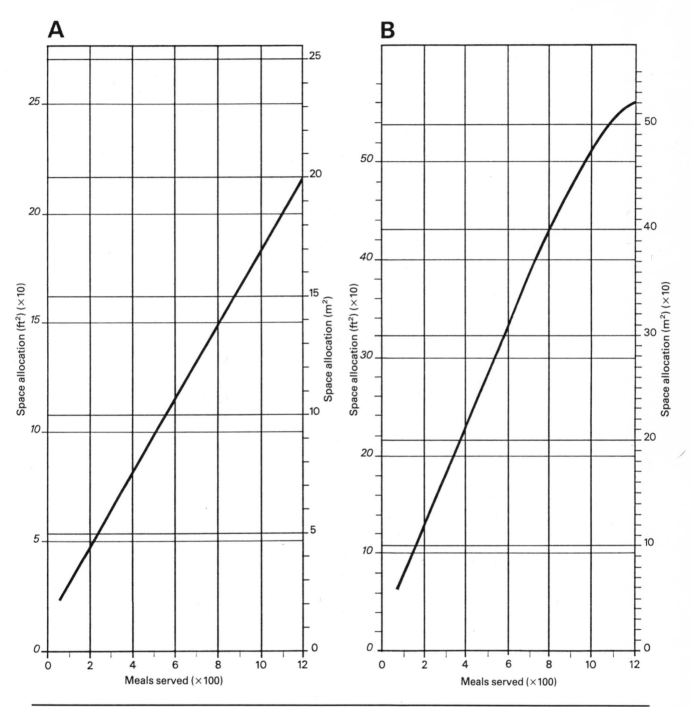

A

Space allocation (ft²) (×10) · Space allocation (m²)

Meals served (×100)

B

Space allocation (ft²) (×10) · Space allocation (m²) (×10)

Meals served (×100)

- In smaller kitchens the potwash area is integrated into the dishwash area to minimize space requirements and maximise the usage of staff.
- In larger facilities (those in excess of 300/400 meals served), mechanical handling systems are used to minimize disruption to the dining area and maximize staff efficiency.

A Graph to show space allocation for potwash.
B Graph to show space allocation for dishwash.

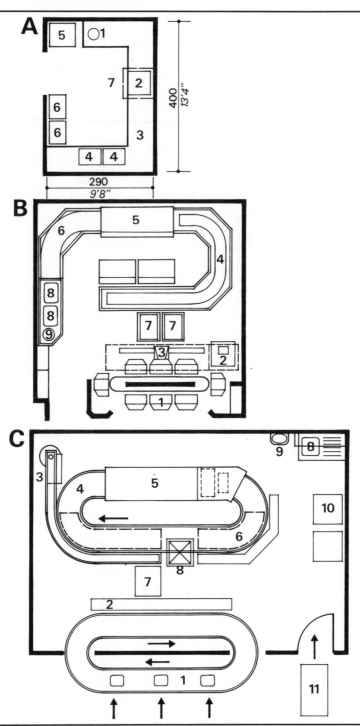

- Circular conveyor makes the system less labor intensive. It is most useful for larger volume operations.
- The dishwash is often separate from the main kitchen to suit customer flow out of the dining area.

A Example of a layout of combined dishwash and potwash for 200 meals.
1 Disposal unit.
2 Dishwasher.
3 Tabling.
4 Sink units, 610mm× 455mm/24″×32″.
5 Tray trolley.
6 Clean crockery trollies.
7 Condense canopy.

B Example of a layout of dishwash for 600 meals.
1 Tray cleaning unit.
2 Scrapping bench.
3 Waste disposal unit.
4 Motorized rack conveyor.
5 Dishwasher.
6 Roller rack conveyor.
7 Bridging tables.
8 Sink unit.
9 Wash-hand basin.

C Example of a layout of dishwash for 1200 meals.
1 Tray cleaning unit.
2 Scrapping bench.
3 Waste disposal unit.
4 Motorised rack conveyor.
5 Dishwasher.
6 Roller rack conveyor.
7 Bridging tables.
8 Sink units.
9 Wash-hand basin.
10 Clean ware.
11 Soiled ware.

1:100

A

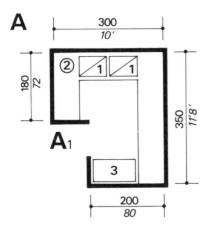

A₁

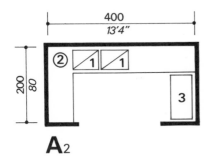

A₂

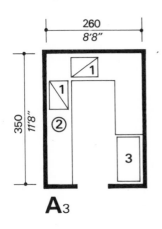

A₃

B

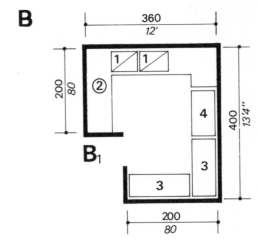

B₁

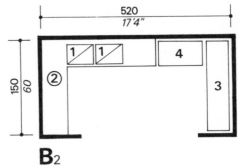

B₂

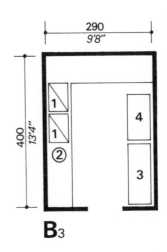

B₃

1:100

A1, A2, A3 Examples of layouts of potwash for 600 meals served.
B1, B2, B3 Examples of layouts of potwash for 1200 meals served.
A 600 meals served.
B 1200 meals served.

1 Sink units, 760×510mm/*30"×20"*.
2 Waste disposal units.
3 Storage racks.
4 Panwashing machine.

COMMERCIAL FOOD PREPARATION
Space allocation: staff facilities,
and cleaning materials storage

2.21

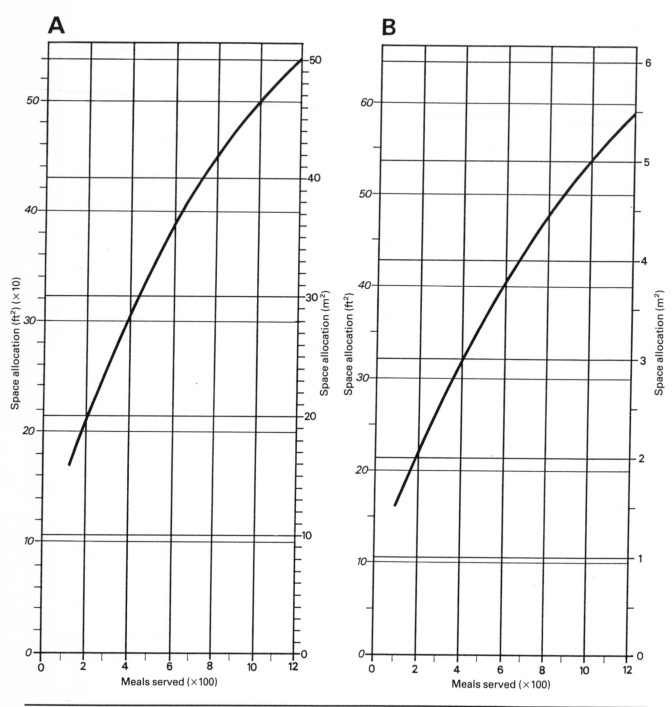

- It is important that good toilet and changing facilities are provided to ensure hygiene standards can be maintained. However, foodservice staff attitudes often reflect the quality of accommodation provided.
- Good staff are more easily retained where washroom and changing facilities are of a high standard.

A Graph to show space allocation for staff facilities.
B Graph to show space allocation for cleaning materials storage.

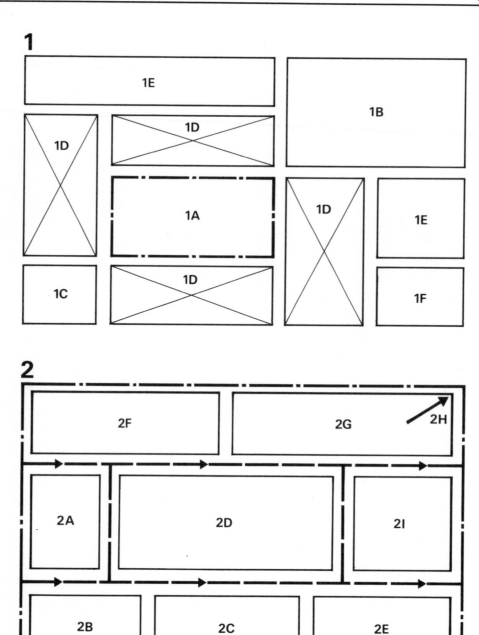

1:100

- Restaurant layout shows the position of the self-service area in relation to seating and kitchen areas.
- Self-service layout shows a possible arrangement within the same area.
- One cashier can serve an average of 6–9 customers per minute, but this depends on the following factors:

a type of cash recovery (till, card swipe).
b whether beverage service is separate.
c whether there are bypass facilities. It is essential to avoid congestion.

1 Restaurant:
1A Bar or self-service area.
1B Kitchen.
1C Entry.
1D Seating.
1E Intimate seating.
1F Washrooms.

2 Self-service:
2A Menu/trays.
2B Starters/soup.
2C Desserts.
2D Salad bar.
2E Drinks/cutlery.
2F Hot/main meals.
2G A la carte (hot assisted).
2H Kitchen.
2I Cash.

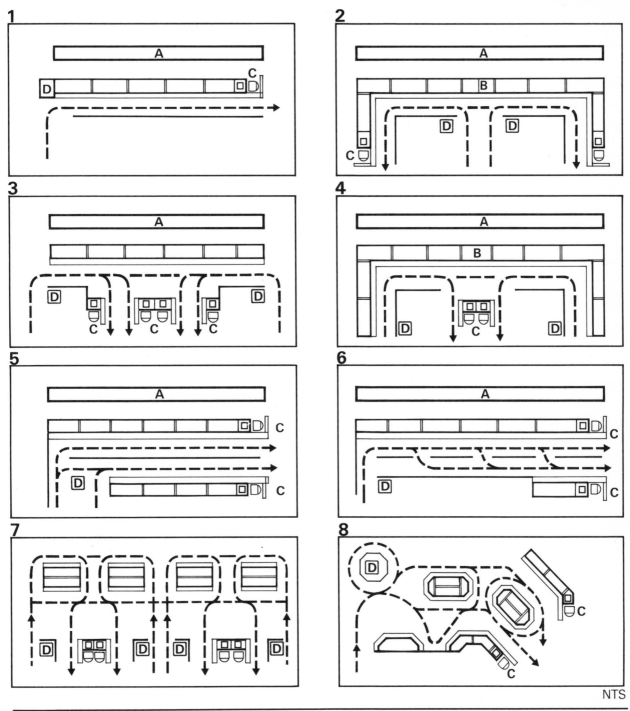

NTS

A Back counter.
B Shared beverages.
C Cash point.
D Trays.

1 Single line: this uses least space. Only one cash point is required.
2 Divergent flow (shared beverage): this doubles the area and menu choice.
3 Multiple outlets allow for a greater number of persons served.
4 Convergent flow with a centralized cash point.
5 Parallel flow permits a greater choice of menu.
6 Bypassing, which allows the customer to go to the cash point once a choice has been made, results in a faster turnover.
7 Free flow (linear): separate servery for each menu classification. Tray slides do not connect, thus avoiding the need to pass all counters.
8 Free flow: separate servery for each menu classification. Tray slides do not connect.

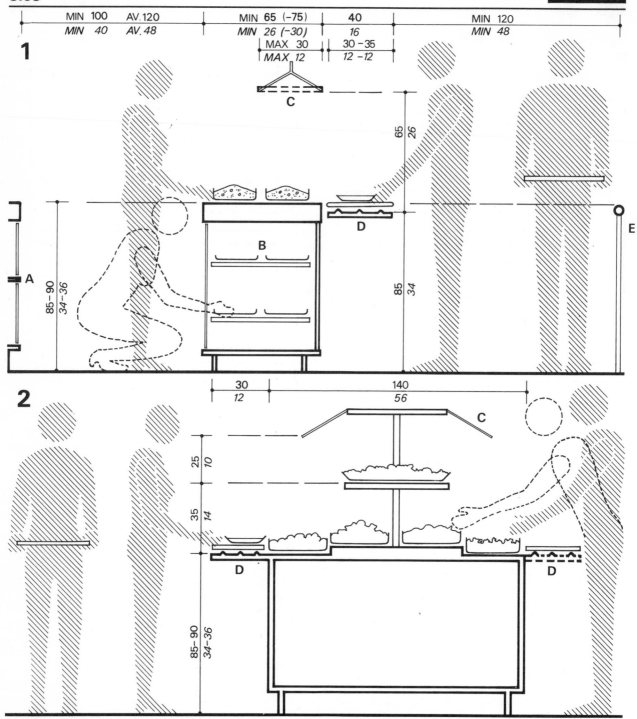

1 Assisted counter service: The customer may take his/her own food or be served. Sufficient room must be left between counters or between the counter and the traffic rail to allow customer flow behind. A sneeze screen is required to protect food.

2 Self-service island unit: allows for separate menus on each island.

A Refrigeration equipment.
B Flat topped serving counter.
C Shelf or glass sneeze screen.
D Tray slide.
E Traffic rail.

3.04

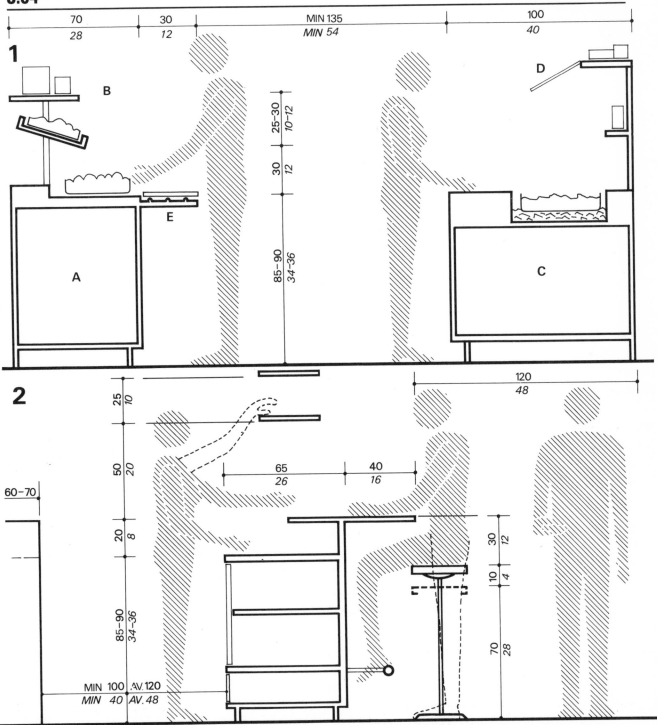

1 Self-service with shelves over.
1A Heated counter with doors to hot cupboard under counter.
1B Glass shelves.
1C Cold counter with tiled recessed area to be filled with ice.
1D Glass sneeze screen.
1E Tray slide: useful for laying trays down while serving. Tray slides do not connect.

2 For counter service (eg bar food, diner): high level shelves should be positioned above eye level.

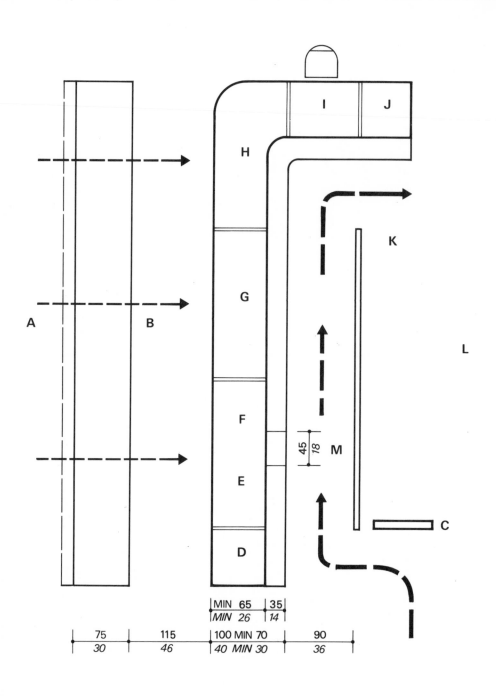

MIN 65 | 35
MIN 26 | 14

75 | 115 | 100 MIN 70 | 90
30 | 46 | 40 MIN 30 | 36

45
18

1:50

- Fewer than 400 customers are served per hour (500–800 in 2½ hours).
- 3m/10' of counter is adequate for every 100 meals served.
- Cold and hot foods are equal in servery length (40–50% of total serving area).
- The customer should spend no more than 5 minutes from the time he/she enters the servery until passing the cash point.

A Kitchen.
B Assisted service.
C Menu.
D Trays.
E Salads.
F Desserts.
G Hot food.
H Drinks.
I Cash point.
J Cutlery.
K Crush rail.
L Seating.
M 45cm zone for 1 customer with tray.

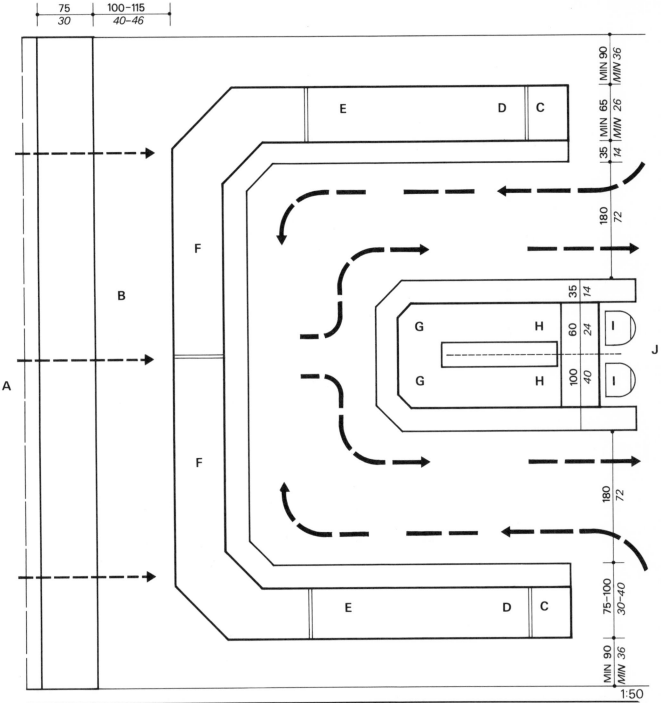

1:50

1000–1500 customers are served in 2½ hours. Total time of approximately 5 minutes is spent as follows:
Tray and utensil selection, 60 sec.
Menu selection, 70 sec.
Salads, entrée, side order selection, 80 sec.
Drink selection, 70 sec.
Travel to cash point, waiting and paying, 60 sec.

A Kitchen.
B Assisted service.
C Trays.
D Desserts.
E Salads.
F Hot foods.
G Drinks.
H Cutlery.
I Cash point.
J Seating.

SERVING AREAS
Assisted separate serving areas:
full meal at the point of service

3.07

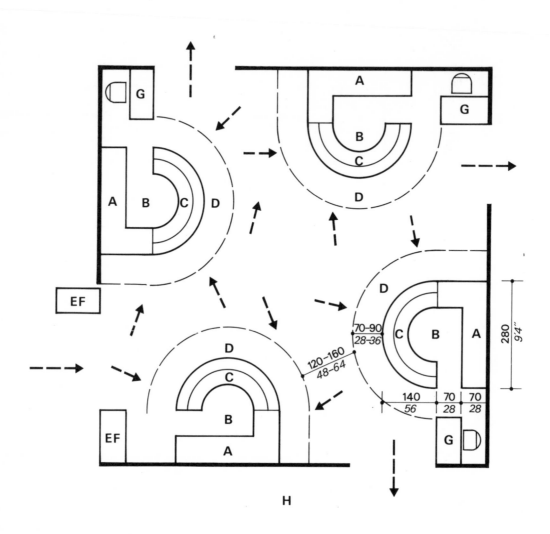

1:100

- The services are free flow.
- Counters are self-sufficient with integrated mini-kitchen (ie regeneration point for pre-cooked/chilled food).
- The system offers wide and varied menus.
- Capacity is limited only by the speed of the cashiers.

A Preparation.
B Full meal.
C Serving area.
D Waiting zone.
E Trays.
F Cutlery.
G Cash point.
H Seating.

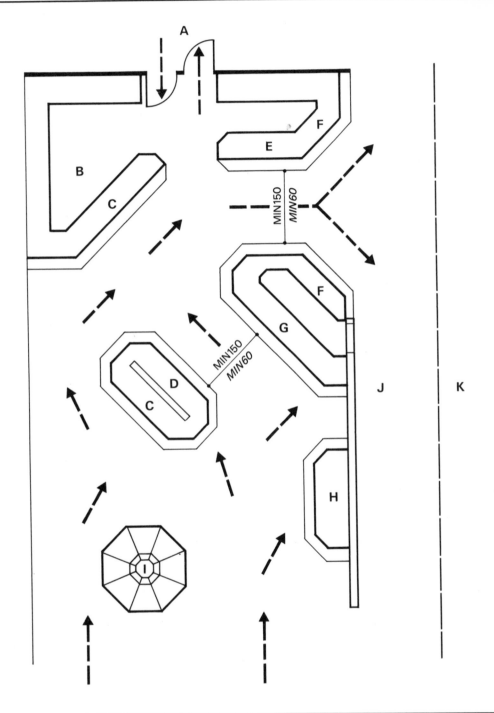

1:100

- The serving areas are free flow.
- The arrangement is comfortable and relaxed.
- Tray slides do not connect counter to counter.
- Customers can change their minds with a minimum of delay.

A Kitchen.
B Assisted service.
C Hot main meal.
D Hot desserts.
E Drinks, cutlery.
F Cash point.
G Cold desserts/cold salads.
H Soup/cold starters.
I Trays.
J Circulation.
K Seating.

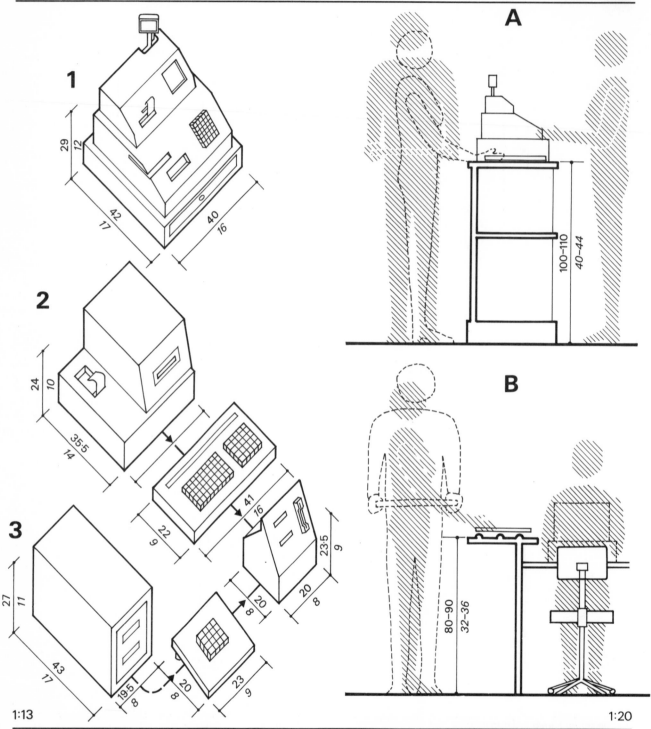

1:13

1:20

A High level register with cashier standing.
B Cashier sitting at 90° to the customer and tray slide. The average rate of serving is 6–9 customers per minute depending on the menu.

1 Standard register/till.
2 Card swipe till.
3 Card swipe mini till.

- Up to 4 customers per minute may be served using credit type cards. Different prices may be charged to different categories of cardholder.
- Mini register: the easiest option where only a small range of items are sold (eg snack bar).

FOOD COURTS
Layout of seating areas, kiosks and
staff support facilities

4.01

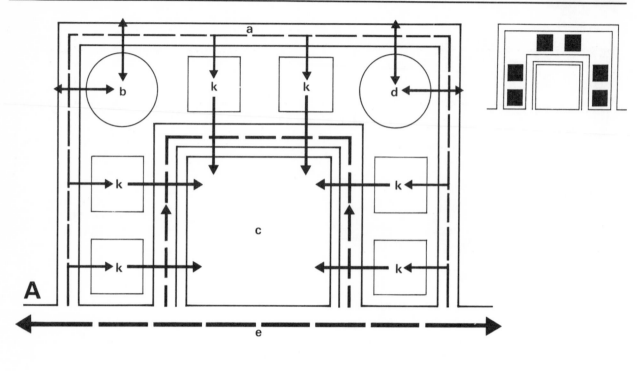

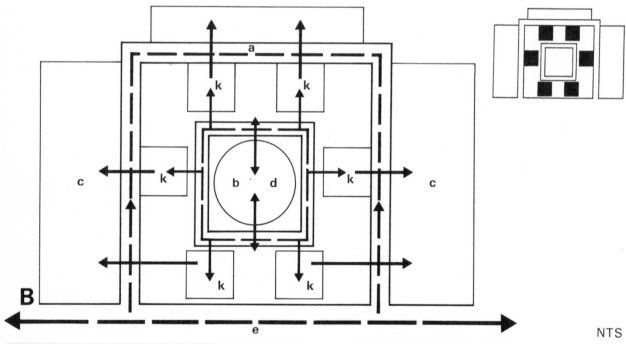

NTS

- Seating is maintained by the operator.
- The customer can choose whichever specialist counter attracts him/her.
- The food court is often located centrally in shopping malls.

A Centralized seating: food court types "L," "U," "linear" and "circular".

B Peripheral seating: food court types "linear" and "circular".

a Service corridor.
b Staff facilities.
c Seating.
d Support facilities.
e Main circulation.
k Kiosk.

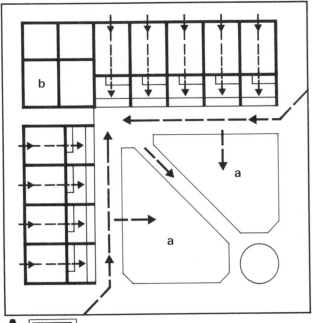

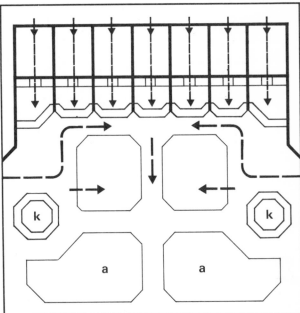

A

B

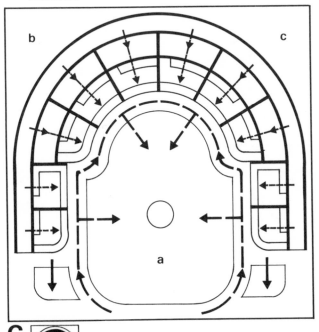

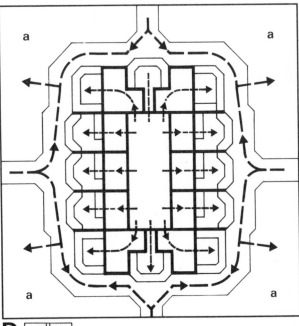

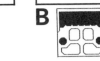

C

D

1:500

- Average number of kiosks is 8–12.
- Average of 40–45 seats per kiosk.
- 50% tenant space and 50% common area.
- 100 seats are positioned over approximately 110m²/ *115 sq yd*, ie 1.1m²/*1.2 sq yd* per seat.

A "L" shaped: optimum traffic flow.
B Linear.
C "U" shaped: optimum traffic flow.
D Circular (exterior seating).

a Seating.
b Washroom
c Refuse.
k Kiosk.

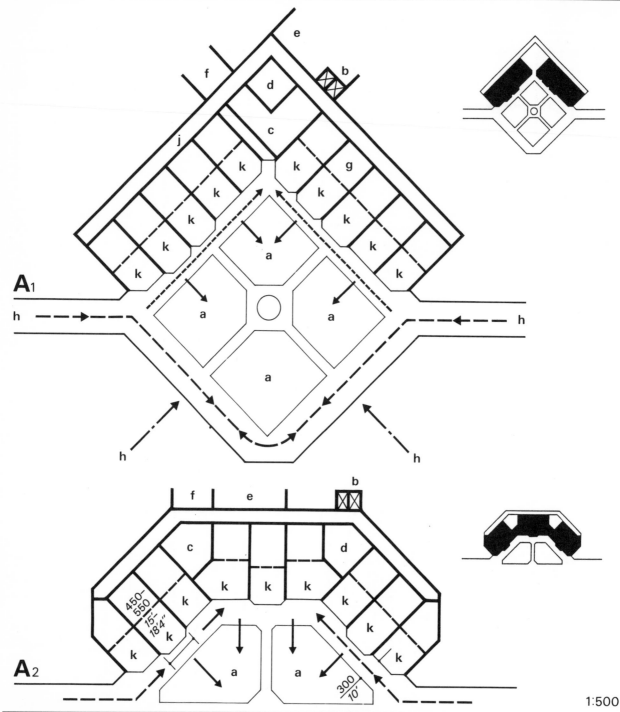

1:500

- Examples of "L" shaped food courts.
- Kiosks are located on 2 sides of the seating area. This arrangement allows for centralized communal areas (eg refuse, stores).
- The advantage is that all kiosks are visible from the malls.

a Seating.
b Service lifts.
c Equipment and crockery storage.
d Refuse.
e Staff toilets and changing area.
f Manager's office.
g Storage area (if required).
h Mall options.
i Circulation.
j Service corridor.
k Kiosks.

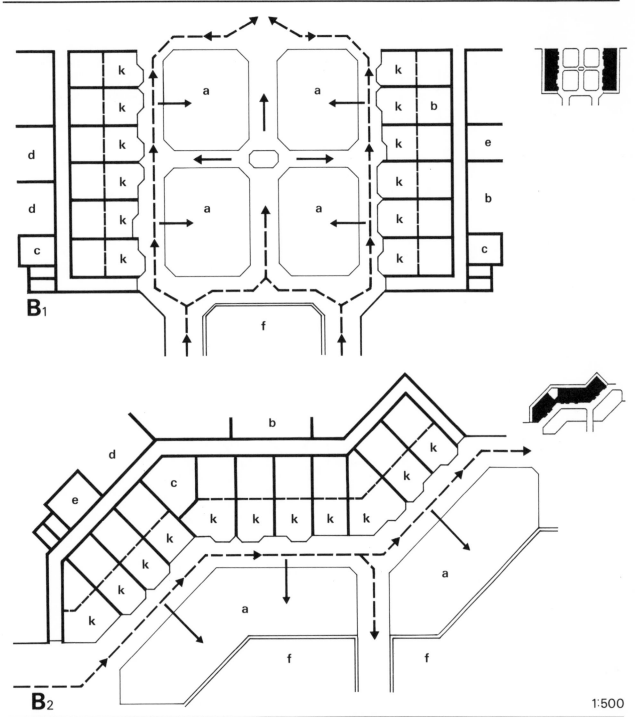

B₁

B₂

1:500

- Examples of linear food courts.
- **B1** When the food court is located so that the customer has to pass through the seating area before moving to another part of the shopping center, this may encourage him/her to buy. The disadvantage is that communal facilities are split.
- **B2** When the kiosks are arranged in one line the customer has to pass all kiosks to see the full choice.

- **a** Seating.
- **b** Storage.
- **c** Refuse.
- **d** Staff washroom.
- **e** Manager's office.
- **f** Space.
- **k** Kiosk.

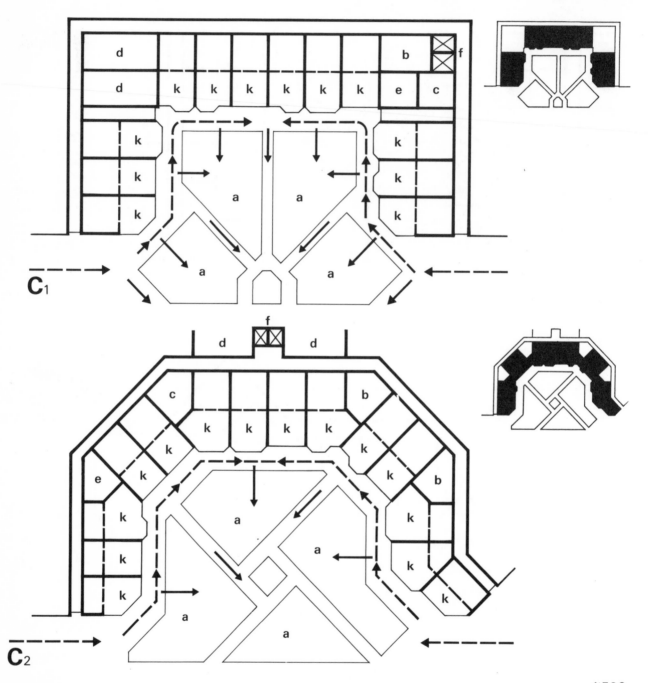

C₁

C₂

1:500

- Examples of "U" shaped food courts. These are similar to "L" shaped but have the advantage of allowing for a greater number of kiosks.
- **C1** Seating for approximately 500.
- **C2** Seating for approximately 600.

a	Seating.
b	**Store.**
c	**Refuse.**
d	Staff washroom and changing facilities.
e	Manager's office.
f	Service lifts.
k	Kiosk.

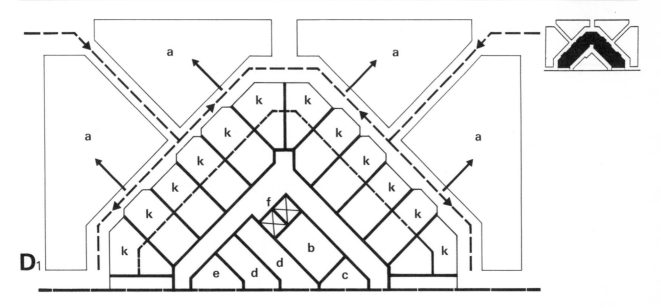

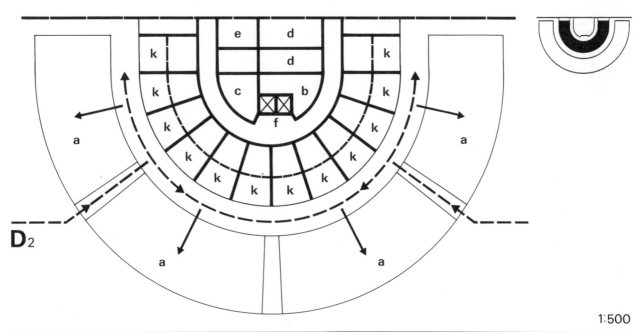

1:500

- Seating is on the periphery of the kiosks.
- The disadvantages of this arrangement are that all kiosks are not visible and the centralized communal facilities result in a "race track" service corridor.

D1, D2 Example of circular/semi-circular type food courts.
a Seating.
b Store.
c Refuse.
d Staff washroom and changing facilities.
e Manager's office.
f Service elevators/lifts.
k Kiosk.

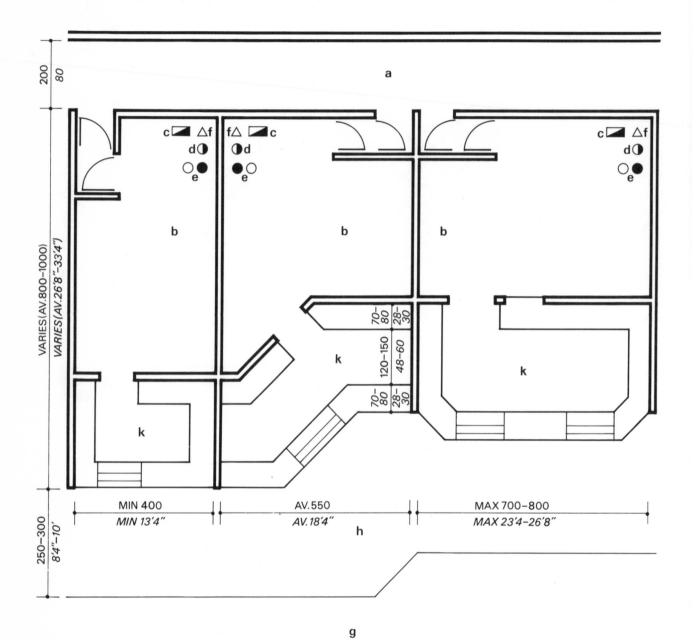

1:100

- Example of a kiosk:
  The average kiosk size is 45–55m²/*54yd²–66yd²*.
  The average frontage is 5–7m/*16'6"–17'8"*.
  The average size of a kiosk with alcohol licence is 100–150m²/*119yd²–179yd²*.
- Services are normally on the back wall.
- Walls and floor are tiled, if possible, for environmental health reasons.

a Service corridor.
b Back-up kitchen and store.
c Extractor/exhaust.
d Gas.
e Hot/cold water.
f Electricity.
   (Incoming services capped-off for tenant connection.)
g Seating.
h Circulation.
k Kiosk.

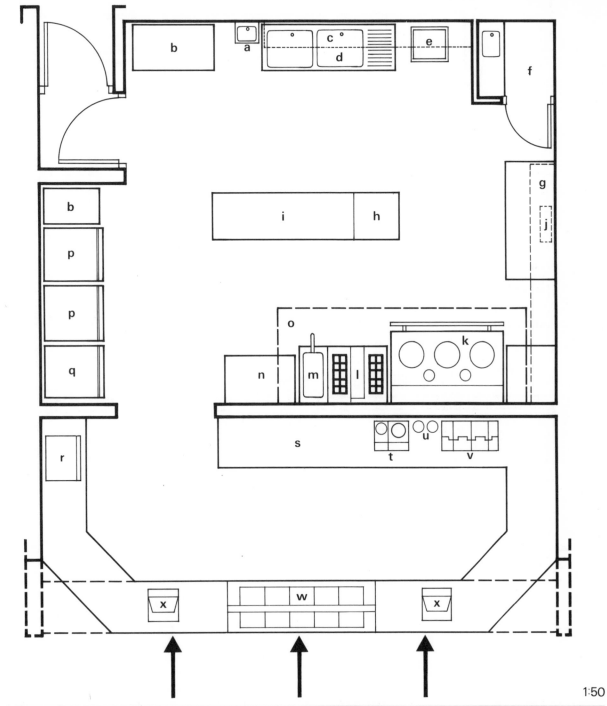

1:50

- Special features of a "Chinese" preparation/serving area:
  Chinese stove, which is especially large allowing 2–3 cooks to work at the same time.
  Central worktop and chopping block.

a Hand basin.
b Storage racks.
c Wall/shelf over.
d Sink unit.
e Mobile refuse.
f Cleaning store and sink.
g Worktop with shelf over.
h Chopping block.
i Central worktop.
j Fly killer/high level.
k Chinese cooker.
l Oven range.

m Fryer.
n Worktop.
o Hood over all cooking.
p Refrigerator.
q Freezer.
r Microwave.
s Back counter.
t Coffee.
u Cups.
v Sodas and juices.
w Hot display.
x Cash point.

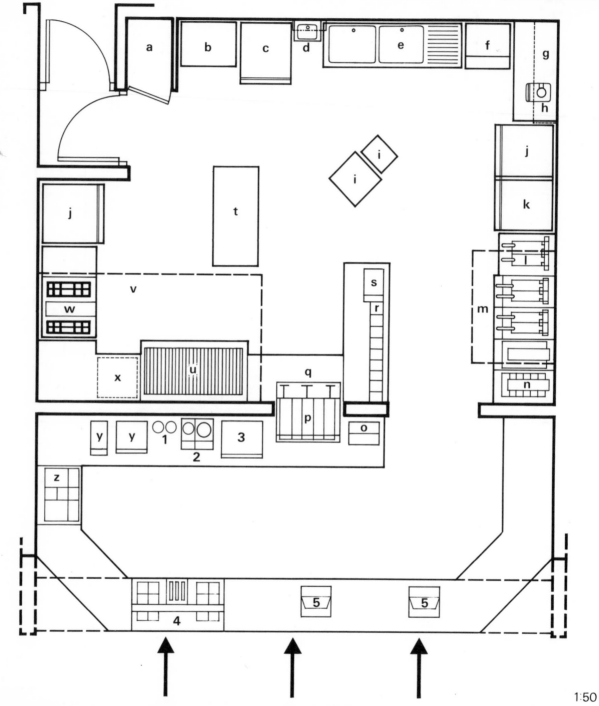

1:50

- Special features of a "Grill" preparation/ serving area:
  Char broilers
  Bench with garnish rack
  Burger chute
  Several fryers and a French fry dump.

a Cleaning store.
b Storage racks.
c Refrigerator.
d Hand basin with fly kill over.
e Sink unit.
f Ice maker.
g Worktop with shelf over.
h Vegetable preparation machine.
i Mobile trolleys.
j Freezer.

k Refrigerator.
l Frying suite.
m Cooker with hood over.
n French fry dump.
o Hot dog display.
p Burger chute.
q Burger wrapping.
r Bench with garnish rack.
s Toaster.
t Mobile central bench.
u Char broilers.
v Stove hood.
w Oven range.

x Mobile burger freezer under worktop.
y Juice and milk.
z Bain marie.
1 Cups.
2 Coffee.
3 Microwave.
4 Hot display with grill.
5 Cash point.

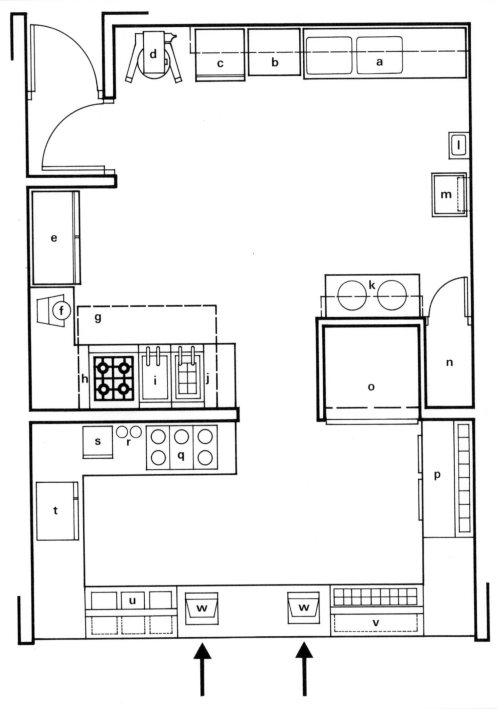

1:50

- Special features of an "Italian" preparation/serving area:
  Mixer
  Refrigerated pizza make-up unit with garnish rack
  Pizza oven.

a	Sink unit with shelf over.
b	Racking.
c	Freezer.
d	Mixer.
e	Refrigerator.
f	Pasta machine on worktop.
g	Stove hood.
h	Oven range.
i	Fryer.
j	Pasta cooker.
k	Worktop with bins and shelf over.

l	Hand basin.
m	Mobile refuse with fly kill over.
n	Cleaning store.
o	Pizza oven.
p	Refrigerated pizza make-up unit with garnish rack.
q	Coffee.
r	Cups.
s	Juice/milk.
t	Microwave.
u	Hot display.
v	Heated tiled display.
w	Cash point.

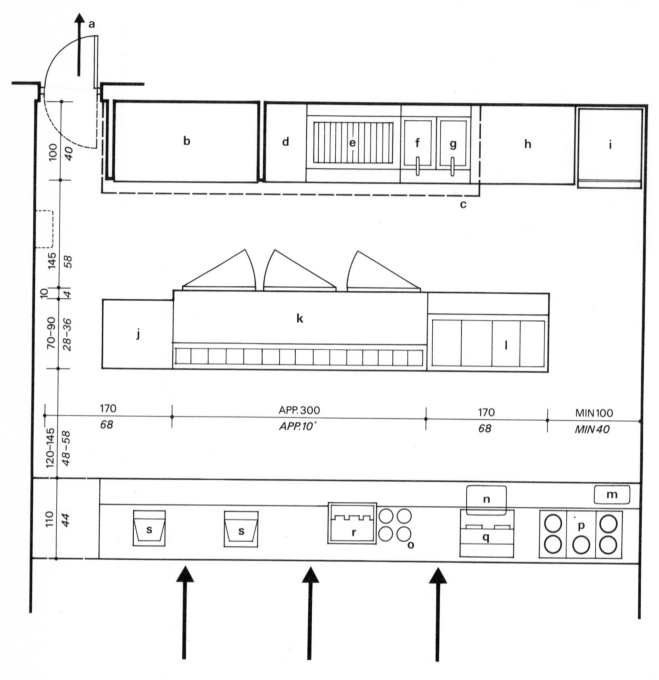

1:50

- Special features of a "Pizza" preparation/serving area:
  Pizza make-up table with garnish racks.
  Pizza oven.

a	To storage.
b	Pizza oven.
c	Stove extract hood.
d	Hot pizza landing.
e	Griddle.
f	Fryer.
g	Fry dump.
h	Worktop.
i	Refrigerator/freezer.
j	Hot pizza landing.
k	Pizza make-up table with storage under and garnish racks.

l	Other hot foods table (optional).
m	Hand basin.
n	Sink.
o	Cups.
p	Coffee.
q	Ice cream.
r	Sodas dispenser.
s	Cash point.

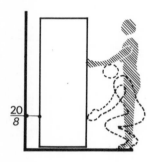
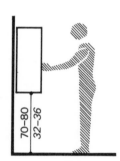
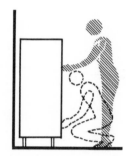
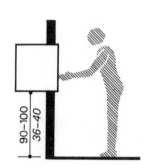

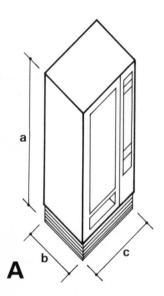

A

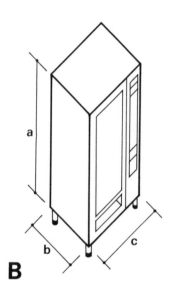

B

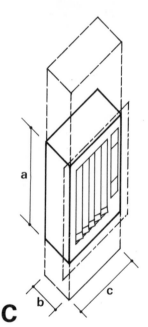

C

1:50

- Refrigerated vending machines require a space of approximately 200mm/8" behind for cooling.
- Service access is generally from the front.
- No hot water supply is required. Some drinks units require a cold water supply with a shut-off valve. The overflow waste falls into an internal bucket or tray.

A Floor mounted with kick plate (type F).
B Floor mounted with legs (type F).
C Wall mounted with "banking" kit (T or B) (type W).

FOOD VENDING UNITS	TYPE	APPROXIMATE DIMENSIONS (mm/in)								
		AVERAGE			MINIMUM			MAXIMUM		
		a (height)	b (depth)	c (width)	a (height)	b (depth)	c (width)	a (height)	b (depth)	c (width)
COLD DRINKS	F	180/72	60/24	97/39	140/56	55/22	70/28	200/80	75/30	115/46
	W	90/36	27/11	70/28	90/36	27/11	70/28	–	–	–
HOT DRINKS	F	180/72	77.5/31	97/36	180/72	68/27	60/24	180/72	85/34	97/36
COLD FOODS	F	180/72	77.5/31	90/36	180/72	76/30	90/36	180/72	90/36	105/42
SWEETS PASTRIES SNACKS	F	180/72	90/36	85/34	180/72	77.5/31	70/28	180/72	90/36	100/40
	W	60/24	60/24	60/24	60/24	60/24	60/24	–	–	–

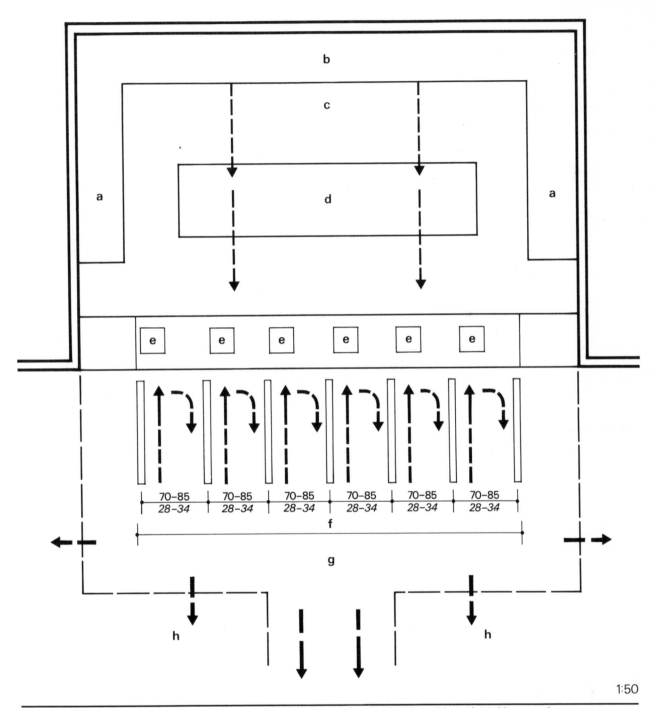

1:50

a Drinks/side orders.
b Preparation.
c Kitchen area (25–30% of total).
d Pre-serve area.
e Cash point.
f Counter (optimum length 8.5m/*9 yd* based on 10 lanes).
g Line up area (20% of total).
h Seating (30–35% of total).

Fast food outlet: with seating/without seating

	% of total area
Kitchen	25–30%/45%
Ancillary (store/washroom)	20%/45%
Space for lines	20%/10%
Seating	30–35%/–

Seating: 1.1m²/*12ft²* per person or 0.5m²/*5ft²* per person with seating ledges.

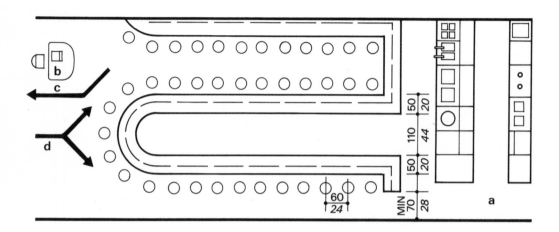

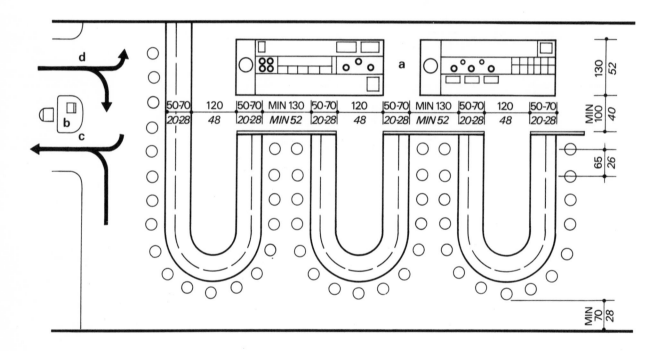

1:100

- Examples of diner/snack bars.
- Areas required:
  1.5–2.15m²/16ft²–23ft² gross per seat.
  Ratio of service area to total area = 25–50%.
  Net kitchen area = 15–25%.
  Kitchen comprises: serving area, cooking, cold buffet,
  preparation and washing up.

a Kitchen.
b Cash point.
c Customers out.
d Customers in.

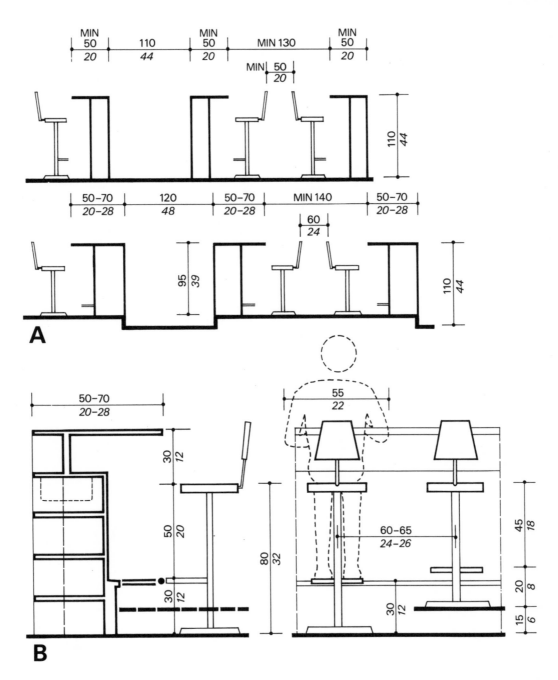

A

B

1:50 /:20

A   Examples of diner/snack bar seating.
B   Customer seated at diner/snack bar.

- 7m–7.5m/7yd² –8yd² length of counter may be served by 1 waiter if meals are pre-cooked.
- Additional 1–2 waiters may be required if meals/drinks are prepared.
- The average sitting time is 20 min.

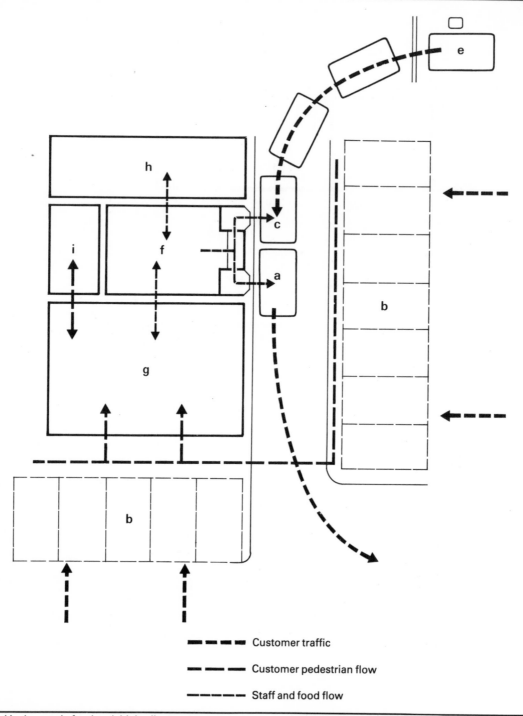

- - - - - Customer traffic

— — — Customer pedestrian flow

— - — - Staff and food flow

NTS

- Drive-in kiosks supply food and drinks direct to cars so that customers may eat without leaving their cars.
- The kiosk forms part of the main kitchen and is served by it.
- For left-hand drive cars this kiosk has to be handed.
- Allow for line up space between "order" and kiosk and before "order".
- Turnover and time spent in line depends on the serving speed.

a Customer serve, position 1.
b Customer parking.
c Customer serve, position 2.
d Microphone order point.
e Stop to order.
f Kitchen.
g Serving area and seating.
h Stores and washroom.
i Customer washroom.

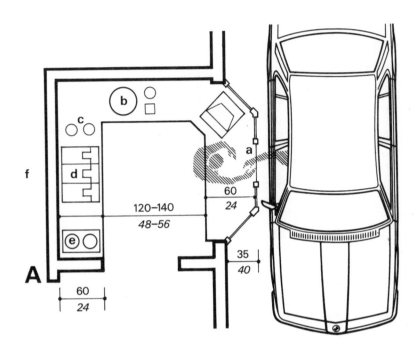

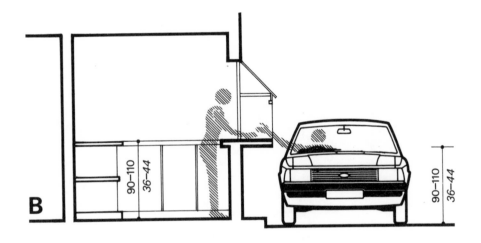

1:50

A Plan view of drive-in kiosk with window service.
B Sectional view of drive-in kiosk with window service.

a Service and cash projecting bay window.
b Soup.
c Cups and lids.
d Juices.
e Coffee.
f Main kitchen.

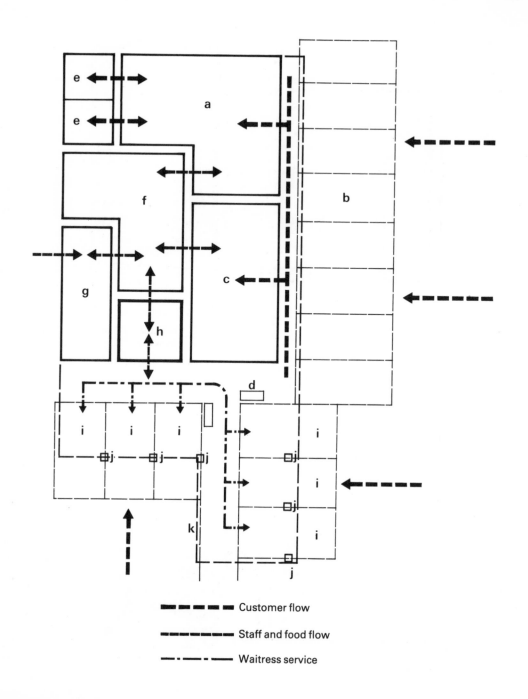

Customer flow

Staff and food flow

Waitress service

NTS

1 Drive-in kiosk serving the same menu as the inside operation. The kiosk is connected to the kitchen.
2 Waitress service from the kiosk to the car.
3 Optional microphone call points.
4 Canopies over walkways.

a Self-service restaurant.
b Parking.
c Snack bar.
d Tray collection point.
e Customer washrooms.
f Kitchen.
g Stores and staff washroom.
h Drive-in kiosk.
i Drive-in car park spaces.
j Microphone call point (optional).
k Canopy.

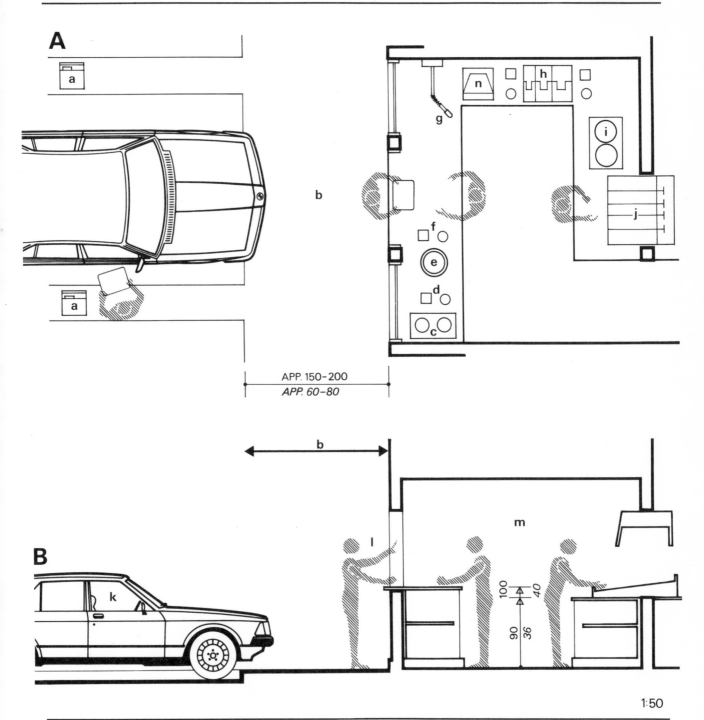

APP. 150–200
APP. 60–80

1:50

- Cooking is carried out in the main kitchen.
- Drinks and dispensers are within the kiosk.
- The waitress delivers food to car/customer and collects when the customer has completed.
- **A** Plan view of drive-in kiosk with waitress service.
- **B** Sectional view of drive-in kiosk with waitress service.

a	Microphone call point (optional).
b	Serving zone (canopy over).
c	Coffee.
d	Cups and lids.
e	Soup well.
f	Bowls and lids.
g	Microphone.
h	Juices.
i	Warming lamps and hot plate.
j	Burger chute.
k	Customer.
l	Waitress.
m	Service.
n	Cash point.

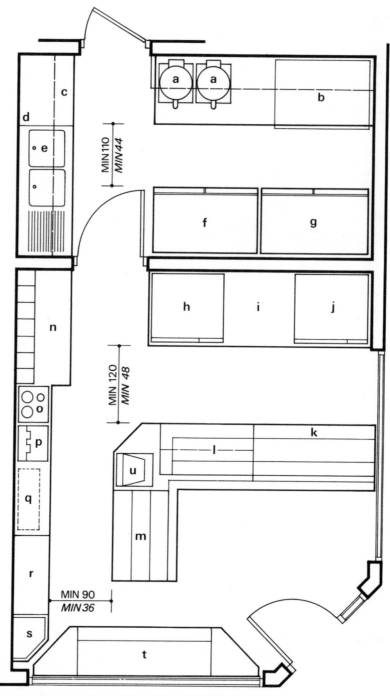

MIN 110 / *MIN 44*

MIN 120 / *MIN 48*

MIN 90 / *MIN 36*

1:50

1 In a small patisserie a certain quantity of baking is done on the premises.
2 Half-baked bread, etc., is delivered from the "central" kitchen.

a Dough mixers.
b Double prover below worktop.
c Worktop.
d Storage over.
e Sink.
f Refrigerator.
g Freezer.
h Prover with oven under.
i Worktop and racks.
j Oven with racks under.
k Hot display counter.

l Display counter.
m Cool display counter.
n Worktop with garnish rack for sandwiches.
o Coffee.
p Milk/juice.
q Bread shelves with basket for French sticks.
r Bread shelves.
s French stick baskets.
t Refrigeration unit for window display.
u Cash point.

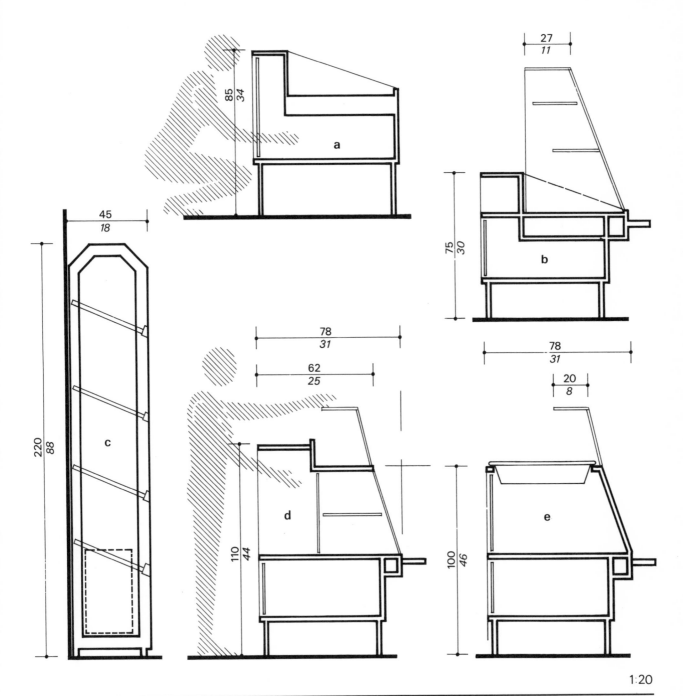

1:20

- Different types of display counter are used for varying patisserie items.
- Hot and refrigerated displays are required.
- Racking is necessary for bread.

a Refrigeration unit for window display.
b Cool display counter with glass shelves.
c Bread shelves with a basket for French sticks.
d Display counter with a glass sliding door.
e Hot display counter with sliding doors, hot plate and glass screen.

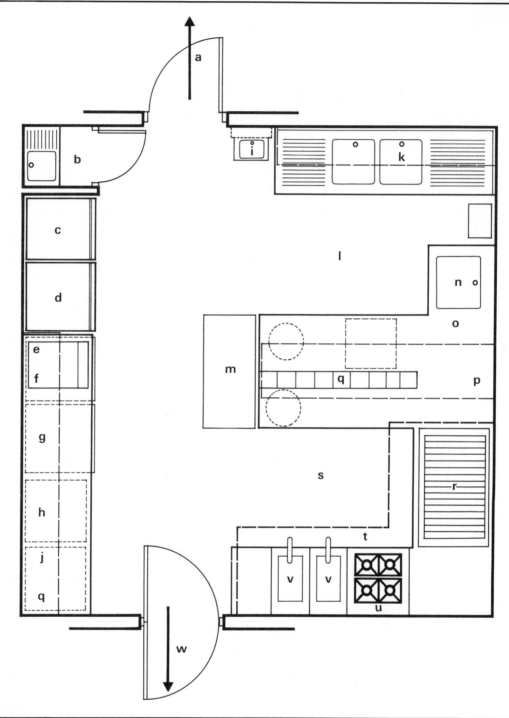

1:50

- Specialized equipment includes: char broiler, garnish table and rack, refrigerators and freezers, stainless steel work surfaces.
- Separate dry storage areas and refuse required.
- Separate pot-wash/dishwash area is desirable if space is available.

a	To storage
b	Cleaners store/cupboard.
c	Large refrigerator.
d	Large freezer.
e	Ice maker.
f	Small refrigerator under worktop.
g	Small freezer under worktop.
h	Mobile rack under worktop.
i	Wash hand basin.
j	Racking.
k	Sink.

l	Vegetable preparation.
m	Mobile bench.
n	Vegetable preparation sink.
o	Worktop.
p	Shelves over.
q	Garnish rack.
r	Char broiler.
s	Grill.
t	Stove hood.
u	Oven range.
v	Fryers.
w	To restaurant seating.

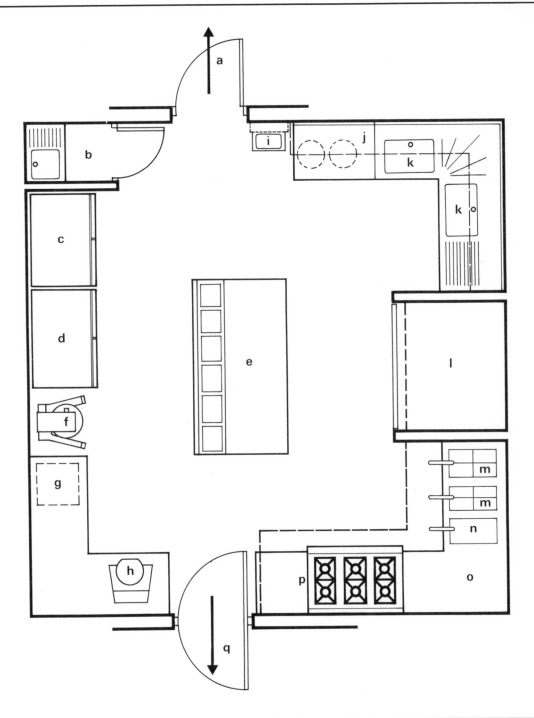

1:50

- Italian restaurant specializing in pasta and pizza with special menu of steak or similar.
- Size of pizza oven vary between 1m×1.5m/*3'3"×5'*.
- Pizza oven requires separate flue over to outside air. Modern pizza ovens have automatic conveyor track set on a timer to bring out pizzas when cooked.
- Dry storage and refuse at back; service room required.

a To storage.
b Cleaners' store and sink.
c Double freezer.
d Double refrigerator.
e Worktop and garnish rack.
f Mixer.
g Worktop with mobile refuse.
h Pasta machine.
i Wash hand basin and fly killer over.

j Worktop with bins under.
k Double sink.
l Pizza oven.
m Pasta cookers.
n Fryer.
o Worktop.
p Stove with oven and hood over.
q To restaurant seating.

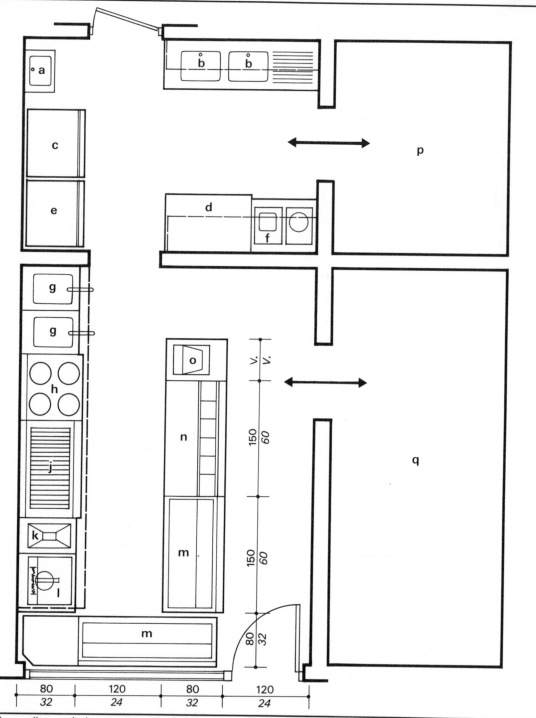

80 / 32   120 / 24   80 / 32   120 / 24

1:50

- If there is an adjacent sit-down restaurant, a larger back-up kitchen will be required, to include additional worktops, oven range, freezer and refrigerator, and wash-up facilities.
- Cold displays are used as storage for skewered meat, salads, desserts and drinks.

a Wash-hand basin.
b Double sink with shelves over.
c Freezer.
d Worktop and chopping table.
e Cold store.
f Mixer and mincer.
g Fryers.
h Oven range.
i Hood over cooking area.
j Griddle with shelves under.

k Bain marie.
l Donner kebabs.
m Cold display.
n Make-up tables with relishes.
o Cash point.
p Back-up kitchen and storage.
q Additional seating area if width of shop is more than 4m/13ft.

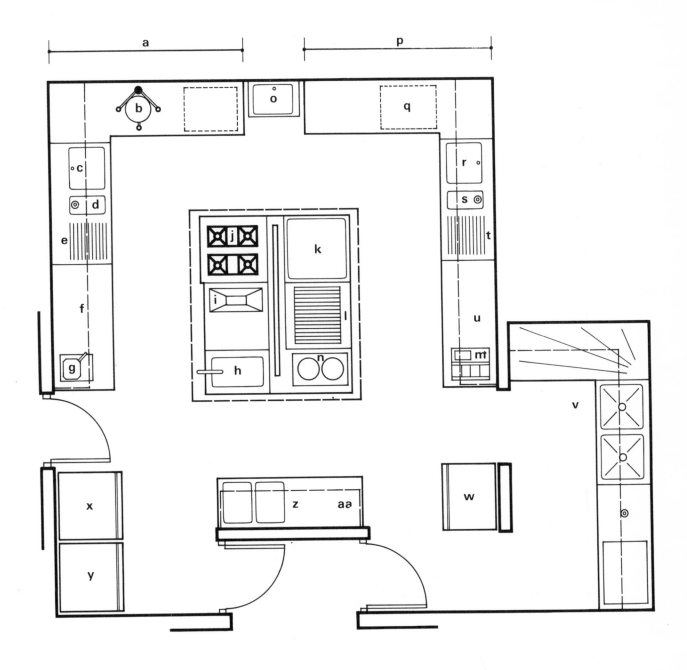

1:50

- Preparation of milk/fish and meat dishes is totally separate.
- A dry store/pantry can be adjacent to the kitchen. Ideally shelves should be slate or stainless steel.
- Passover cupboard should contain separate pots and crockery for use only for passover meal.
- The wash-up facility is communal for both milk/fish and meat dishes.

a	Milk/fish preparation.
b	Mixer on worktop.
c	Sink.
d	Waste disposal.
e	Drain.
f	Storage over.
g	Kettle.
h	Fryer.
i	Bain marie.
j	Oven range.
k	Convection oven.
l	Grill shelves under.
m	Slicer.
n	Hotplates.
o	Wash hand basin.

p	Meat preparation.
q	Mobile rack under worktop.
r	Sink.
s	Waste disposal.
t	Drain.
u	Storage under and over.
v	Wash-up.
w	Meat refrigerator.
x	Milk/fish refrigerator.
y	Freezer.
z	Pre-serve worktop with hotplates.
aa	Passover cupboard over.

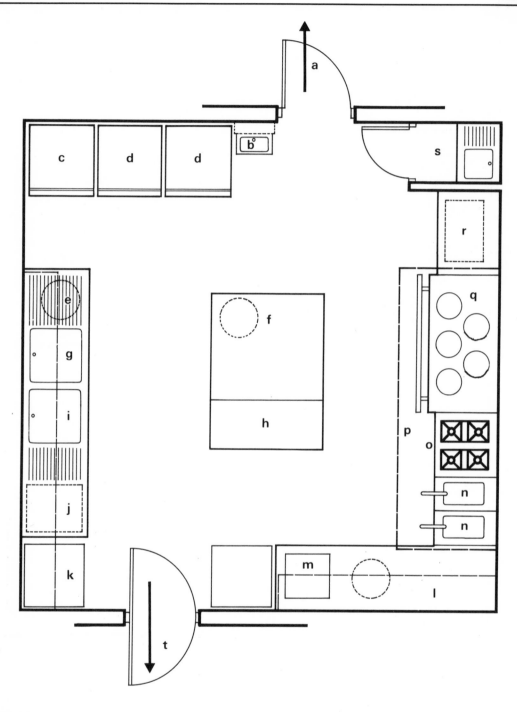

1:50

- It is essential to have long lengths of worktops with refuse bins under.
- Space around the Chinese stove is required so that several cooks may work at the cooker at the same time.
- Sink is mainly used for food preparation.
- Additional sinks are required for wash-up.
- Additional dry store is required.

a To storage.
b Wash hand basin and fly killer over.
c Freezer.
d Refrigerator.
e Refuse under.
f Central worktop with refuse.
g Double sink.
h Chopping block.
i Shelving over.
j Mobile rack under worktop.

k Racking.
l Worktop with shelves over.
m Rice steamer.
n Fryers.
o Oven range.
p Hood over.
q Chinese stove.
r Worktop with mobile rack.
s Cleaners' store/ cupboard.
t To restaurant seating.

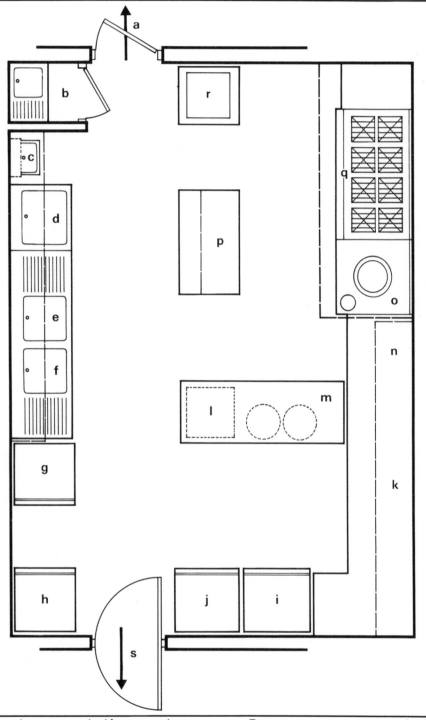

1:50

- Long lengths of worktops are required for preparation of dishes.
- Double sink and drainer is used both for food preparation and dishes wash-up.
- Deep sink is used for dishes and pot wash.
- Specialist items include a tandoori oven and large oven range and rice steamer.

a	To store.
b	Cleaners' store/cupboard.
c	Wash-hand basin and fly killer over.
d	Deep sink.
e	Shelves over.
f	Double sink and drainer.
g	Low refrigerator.
h	High refrigerator.
i	High freezer.

j	High refrigerator.
k	Pot store under.
l	Mobile rack.
m	Worktop (bins under).
n	Worktop and shelves over.
o	Tandoori oven.
p	Worktop.
q	Oven range.
r	Rice steamer.
s	To restaurant seating.

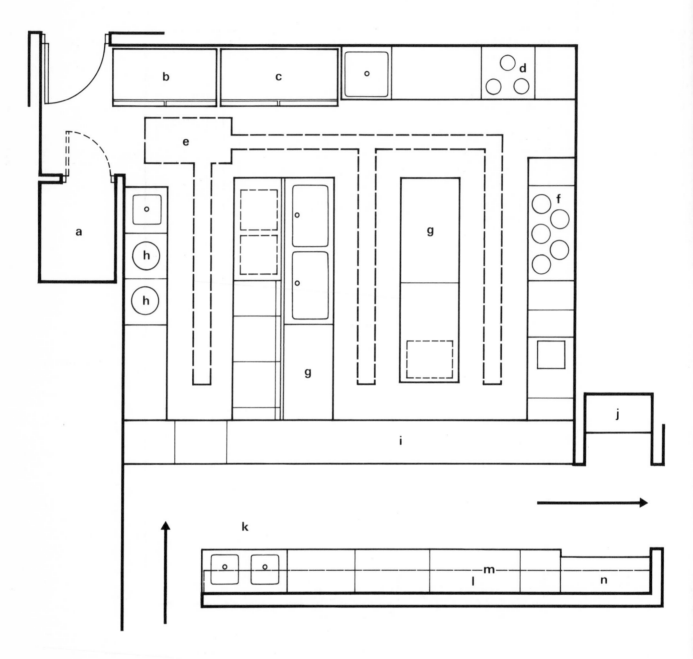

1:50

- Traditional kitchen includes a pantry for laying out food prior to distribution to tables.
- Special items to be included: iron pots ("Sobagama") for noodles, large gas oven, hot plates.
- Storage (dry) is outside main kitchen.
- Drink storage is in the pantry area.

a	Cleaners' store.
b	Refrigerator.
c	Freezer.
d	Hot plates.
e	Vent extractor/exhaust at high level.
f	Gas oven.
g	Work top.
h	Iron pots, "Sobagama" (noodles).

i	Service counters.
j	Ice machine.
k	Pantry.
l	Beer cooler.
m	Shelves over.
n	Shelves.

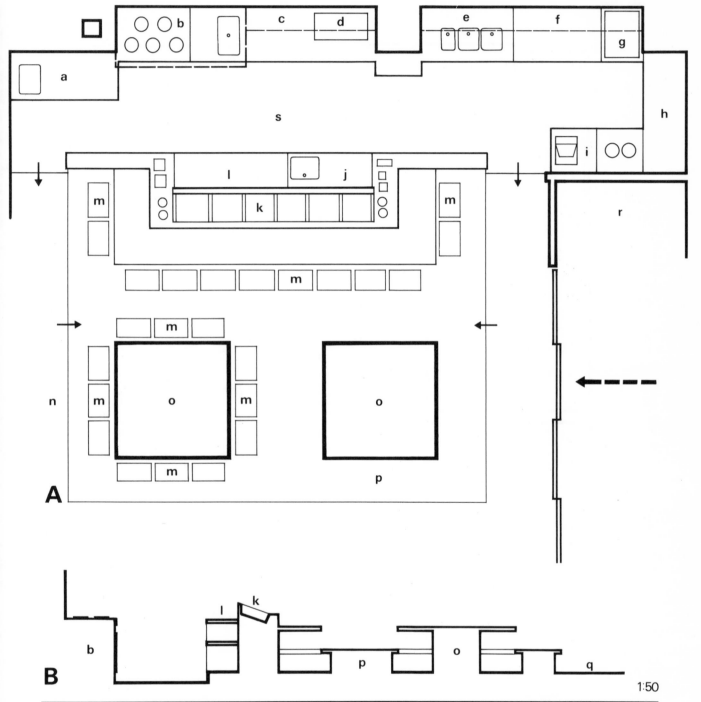

1:50

A Plan view of Japanese-style diner.	**a** Worktop and sink.	**k** Food display.
B Sectional view of Japanese-style diner.	**b** Stove with hood.	**l** Sandwich table.
• This type of diner has a raised platform for seating and lowered kitchen area with large communal tables.	**c** Worktop with shelves over.	**m** Cushions.
		n Bench seating.
• Additional bench seating is provided around the periphery.	**d** Beer cooler.	**o** Big pine table.
• Food display is prominent on the front counter.	**e** Wash-up sink.	**p** Pine board floor (+30/12).
	f Worktop.	**q** Passage (±0).
• Snacks and sandwiches are prepared at the front counter.	**g** Ice maker.	**r** Washroom.
	h Store.	**s** Kitchen (−15/6).
Note: It is traditional that shoes are removed for diners sitting on the raised platform.	**i** Cash point.	
	j Worktop.	

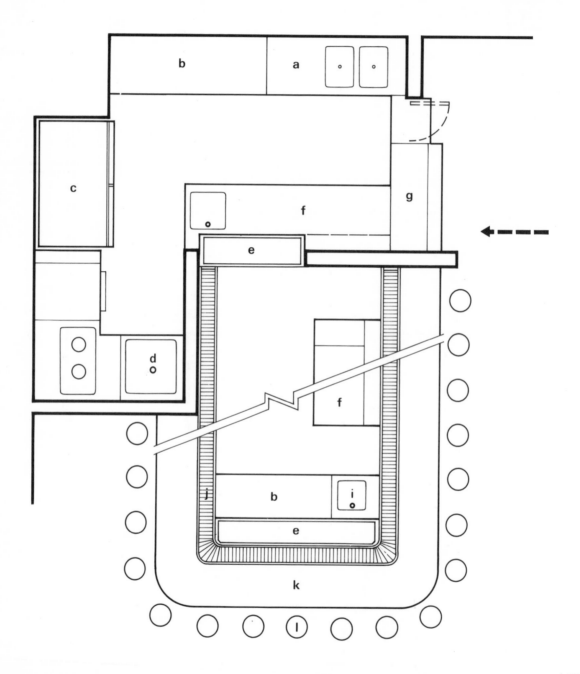

1:50

- This type of "sushi" bar has a moving conveyor for distribution of "sushi" to customers seated on bar stools around the counter.
- The counter length can vary depending on the size of spaces.
- Kitchen area is small – for storage of "sushi" and preparation. There is a small sink for washing dishes.
- The display counter is located at the entrance to enable customers to make their choice as they enter.

a   Wash-up sink.
b   Worktop.
c   Refrigerator/freezer.
d   Sink.
e   Display case.
f   Preparation.
g   Display table.
h   Bowls and sauce beneath conveyor.
i   Sink.
j   "Sushi" conveyor.
k   Counter.
l   High stools.

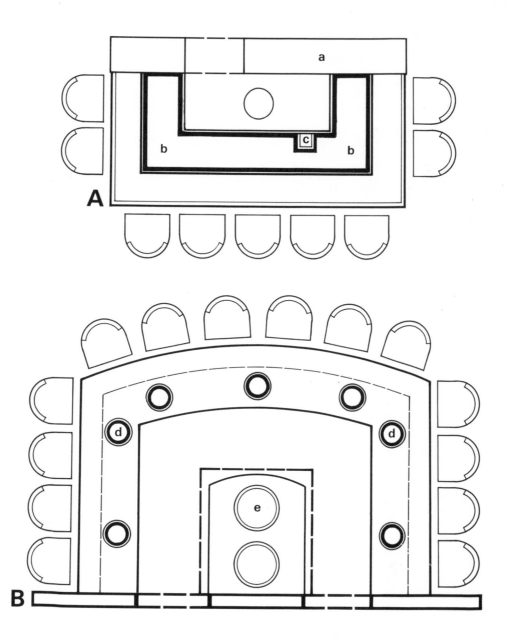

1:50

A Steak counter: Cooking is carried out at the table by the cook (e.g. beihana). The hotplate has varying degrees of heat over the total area. There is a waste chute to refuse bin below.

B Barbecue: Charcoal is heated in the central fireplace and distributed to the charcoal containers for individual cooking by customers. Two customers share one container.

a Back counter for relishes, sauces, etc.
b Hot plate with varying degrees of heat.
c Waste.
d Individual charcoal containers (fed from main fireplace).
e Charcoal fireplace with extractor/hood hood over.

BIBLIOGRAPHY

Baratan, Regina S/Durocher, Joseph F. (Ph.D.): *Successful Restaurant Design,* 1988.
De N. Sairoedner, Francis: *Anatomy for Interior Designs (2nd Edition) and How to talk to a Client.*
Excellent Shop Designs: *Japanese Restaurants and Taverns 2,* 1989.
Firchfield, J.: *Design and Layout Foodservice Facilities,* 1988.
Kazarian, E.: *Foodservice Facilities Planning,* 1988.
Lawson, Fred: *Restaurant Planning and Design,* 1973.
Lawson, Fred: *Principles of Catering Design,* 2nd Edition, 1978.
Medlik, S.: *Profile of the Hotel and Catering Industry,* 1972.
Neufert, E.: *Architects' Data (trans.),* 1980.
Pegler, M.: *Successful Food Merchandising and Display,* 1989.
Prina, Alberto Maria/Bergamasdu, Giovanna: *Kitchen, Cooking and Culture, From the Stove to the Computer, A Route Towards the Year 2000,* Milan, 1984.
Ramsey, C. G./Sleeper, H. R.: *Architectural Graphic Standards,* 8th ed., New York, 1988.
Scriven, C. and Stevens, J.: *Manual of Equipment and Design for the Foodservice Industry,* 1989.
Wilkinson, Julie: *The Anatomy of Foodservice Design 1,* 1975.
Wilkinson, Julie: *The Anatomy of Foodservice Design 2,* 1978.
Food Counts – How to Develop a Food Count in Your Shopping Centre, International Council of Shopping Centres 1987.
New Metric Handbook: Planning and Design Data, Reprinted 1985.
Designers Journal 1986–1989.

Product manufacturers' literature:
AEG
Sie Matic
Smallbone of Devizes
Paggenpohl
Gaggenau
Miele